132 Care Plan Templates

By SHEENA JOHNSTONE

Copyright © 2020 Planning For Care Limited
All rights reserved

Disclaimer

The content of this publication does not constitute advice on which decisions can be based, and it is provided for general information purposes only. Professional or specialist advice should always be sought before taking any action relating to health issues and care plans. Insofar as is permitted by law, we make no representation, warranty, or guarantee that the content of this publication will meet your requirements, that it will not infringe the rights of third parties, that it will be compatible with all cases, or that it will be secure. We make reasonable efforts to ensure that the content is complete, accurate, and up-to-date. We do not, however, make any representations, warranties or guarantees (whether express or implied) that the content is complete, accurate, or up-to-date. The author, Sheena Johnstone, and the company, Planning For Care Limited, have no responsibility for any health and economic damage, and the user of this guide bears exclusively the responsibility.

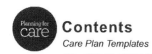

Contents
Care Plan Templates

Introduction	5
Actinic Keratoses	6
Activity and Movement Whilst on Bed Rest	8
Allergy	10
Anaemia Iron Deficiency	12
Angina	14
Anticipatory or Advance	16
Behaviour Agitated Anxious	18
Behaviour Angry or Aggressive	20
Bipolar Disorder	22
Bone Cancer	24
Bowel Cancer	26
Bowel Polyps	28
Brain Haemorrhage	30
Brain Tumour	32
Breast Cancer	34
Breathing Difficulty	36
Bruise	38
Bullous Pemphigoid	40
Burn or Scald	42
Catheter Care	44
Cellulitis	46
Chest Infection	48
Cholecystitis	50
Chronic Kidney Failure	52
Chronic Lymphocytic Leukaemia	54
Chronic Urinary Retention	56
Cirrhosis	58
Coeliac Disease	60
Colostomy	62
Common Cold	64
Communication Difficulty	66
Conjunctivitis	68
Constipation	70
Covert Medication Administration	72
Crohn's Disease	74
Deep Vein Thrombosis	76
Dehydration	78
Dementia Alzheimer's Disease	80
Dementia Vascular	82
Dementia with Lewy Bodies	84
Dementia	86
Depression	88
Diabetes	90
Diverticular Disease	92
Dressing and Undressing	94
Dry Skin	96
Ear Infection Outer Ear	98
Earwax	100
Eczema	102
Epilepsy	104
Faecal Incontinence	106
Falls Risk	108
Fibromyalgia	110
Flu	112
Fluid Intake	114
Fractured Ribs	116
Gastroenteritis	118
Generalised Anxiety Disorder	120
Glaucoma	122
Gout	124
Guillain Barré Syndrome	126
Haemorrhoids	128

Heart Attack	130
Heart Failure	132
Heartburn	134
Hepatitis	136
Hernia	138
Hiatus Hernia	140
Huntington Disease	142
Hypertension	144
Hypotension	146
Implantable Cardioverter Defibrillator	148
Irritable Bowel Syndrome	150
Kidney Infection	152
Korsakoffs Syndrome	154
Labyrinthitis Inner Ear Infection	156
Leg Ulcer	158
Lichen Planus	160
Lung Cancer	162
Medication Administration	164
Migraine	166
Mild Cognitive Impairment	168
Mobility and Physical Activity	170
Motor Neurone Disease	172
Moving and Assisting	174
MRSA Positive	176
Multiple Sclerosis	178
Muscle Cramps	180
Muscular Dystrophy	182
Myasthenia Gravis	184
Nutrition Intake	186
Nutritional Intake Inadequate	188
Oral Hygiene	190
Oral Thrush	192
Osteoarthritis	194
Osteoporosis	196
Pacemaker	198
Pain	200
Palliative	202
Parkinson Disease	204
PEG Feed Percutaneous Endoscopic Gastrostomy	206
Pelvic Organ Prolapse	208
Pernicious Anaemia	210
Personal Hygiene	212
Pneumonia	214
Post-Fracture	216
Pressure Area Care	218
Pressure Sore	220
Prostate Cancer	222
Prostate Enlargement	224
Psoriasis	226
Pulmonary Embolism	228
Recreation	230
Rheumatoid Arthritis	232
Schizophrenia	234
Sepsis	236
Shingles	238
Skin Abscess	240
Skin Cancer	242
Sleeping	244
Spirituality	246
Stroke	248
Ulcerative Colitis	250
Underactive Thyroid	252
Unsteady Gait	254
Urinary Incontinence	256
Urinary Tract Infection	258
Vaginal Thrush	260
Validation and Memory Aids	262
Vertigo	264
Visual Impairment	266
Warfarin	268

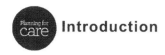

Introduction

This volume consists of a practical guide with 132 different Care Plans for different conditions and medical and health issues.

Aiming at a practical help to other nurses and carers, the primary objectives of this publication focus on:

- Meeting regulators requirements regarding paperwork.
- Creating more time to provide excellent personalised treatment.

Our Care Plans provide a direction on the type of nursing care, the individual, or family and community may need. The main focus is to facilitate standardised evidence-based and holistic approach.

The Care Plans include within it a set of actions the nurse or carer apply to resolve or support nursing diagnosis identified by nursing assessments.

Furthermore, they are personalised to the individual and their needs—support required for the individual, which could include adaptations or equipment to make their life easier.

Dedicated to nurses, key workers and carers, our templates are committed to the highest standards of care to:

- Ensure the production of accurate and detailed nursing care plans.
- Secure all risks are identified and assessed.
- Guide and direct towards the right questions for the determination of the issues the resident faces.
- Help the analysis and the setup of the care plan that is necessary for each resident.
- Provide a useful and detailed explanatory note on each issue, giving valuable information to the person preparing or using the care plan.
- Dramatically reduce time spent preparing and writing care plans.

The care plans should be under review at a minimum of once every 30 days, and, where appropriate, updates require log records.

Last but not least, our Care Plan Templates are easy to use, and this edition adopts the state-of-the-art in digital publishing for full compatibility, functionality, and interactivity across all media platforms and devices.

For more information about our Nursing Care Plans and the available digital downloads, please visit our website at https://www.planningforcare.co.uk/

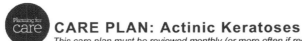

CARE PLAN: Actinic Keratoses

This care plan must be reviewed monthly (or more often if required) and each action must be signed and dated

Actinic keratoses are dry scaly patches of skin caused by damage from years of sun exposure. The patches can be pink, red or brown in colour, and can vary in size from a few millimetres to a few centimetres across. The skin in affected areas can sometimes become very thick, and occasionally the patches can look like small horns or spikes. The patches are usually harmless, but they can be sore, itchy and look unsightly. There is also a risk that the patches could develop into a type of skin cancer called squamous cell carcinoma if they are not treated.

Patient's Issues and Objectives	Consultation Assessment and Plan	Signature	Date	Review Date
Actinic keratoses Promotion and maintenance of healthy skin	1. Discuss the condition with the patient and, or the relative and agree the plan of care.			
	2. Note the patient's and, or relative's understanding of the condition and any concerns or anxieties they have:			
	3. Detail the patient's past history of actinic keratoses:			
	4. Identify the area(s) affected with actinic keratoses:			
	5. Detail the dimensions of the area of skin affected:			
	6. Detail the description of the actinic keratoses and any symptoms experienced: | RED AREA | PINK AREA | BROWN AREA | ROUGH | SCALY | FLAT | RAISED | WART LIKE | SORE | ITCHY | BLEEDING |			
	7. Note the prescribed treatment regime:			
	8. Identify any issues with the application of creams or treatment regime:			

Copyright © 2020 Planning For Care Limited

CARE PLAN: Actinic Keratoses

This care plan must be reviewed monthly (or more often if required) and each action must be signed and dated

Patient's Issues and Objectives	Consultation Assessment and Plan	Signature	Date	Review Date
	9. Liaise with the patient's General Practitioner or dermatologist as necessary.			

Name	Resident/Relative Signature	Date

Copyright © 2020 Planning For Care Limited

CARE PLAN: Activity and Movement Whilst On Bed Rest

This care plan must be reviewed monthly (or more often if required) and each action must be signed and dated

Physical activity, such as regular exercise, is important for health. People who are chronically ill, elderly, or disabled are particularly susceptible to the adverse effects of prolonged bed rest, immobilisation, and inactivity. The detrimental effects of immobility are rarely confined to only one body system. Immobility in the elderly often cannot be prevented, but many of its adverse effects can. When muscles aren't used, they rapidly begin to weaken and waste away. Strength can decrease as much as 20-30% after only a week of complete bed rest, and it generally takes much longer to regain the strength than it took to lose it. Immobility can also lead to limited joint movement. The cartilage around joints begins to deteriorate, while the connective tissue thickens and the muscles shorten, typically at the hip, knee and shoulder. Relatively small regular improvements in mobility or movement can decrease the incidence and severity of complications and improve the well-being of the elderly.

Patient's Issues and Objectives	Consultation Assessment and Plan	Signature	Date	Review Date
Activity and movement whilst confined to bed To promote and encourage participating in movement and activity	1. Discuss the importance of activity and movement with the patient and, or relative and agree the plan of care.			
	2. Note any concerns or anxieties they have:			
	3. Note the reason for bed rest:			
	4. Detail any physical disability or health issues which may restrict the patient's movement:			
	5. Note if the patient has any issues with memory or understanding:			
	6. Note the agreed plan for moving or transferring the patient and the equipment which must be used for the safety of the patient and the nurse or carer:..			
	7. Detail the agreed plan of care for the patient to actively, or passively move limbs, minimising the risk of muscle wasting and contractures:..			

Copyright © 2020 Planning For Care Limited

CARE PLAN: Activity and Movement Whilst On Bed Rest

This care plan must be reviewed monthly (or more often if required) and each action must be signed and dated

Patient's Issues and Objectives	Consultation Assessment and Plan	Signature	Date	Review Date
	8. Detail the agreed plan of care and frequency to support or assist the patient to change position as required:			
	9. Note what type of physical activity the patient would like to, or could take part in whilst in bed:			
	10. Highlight the patient's preference for recreation or mental stimulation:| READING | CROSSWORDS | TELEVISION | | DVDS | RADIO MUSIC | RADIO TALK SHOWS |...............			
	11. Note the patient's preferred choices of television programmes, radio station, or type of music or books:			
	12. Liaise with the patient's General Practitioner, physiotherapist or healthcare worker for advice, as necessary.			

Name	Patient/Relative Signature	Date

Copyright © 2020 Planning For Care Limited

CARE PLAN: Allergy

This care plan must be reviewed monthly (or more often if required) and each action must be signed and dated

An allergy is an adverse reaction, which the body has, or may have, to a particular food or substance in the environment, such as a medicine, pollen, dust mites, pet hair, or foods such as, shellfish and nuts. Allergies occur when the immune system reacts to a foreign substance or allergen as though it is a threat, like an infection. It produces antibodies to fight off the allergen. The next time a person comes into contact with the allergen, the body recalls the previous exposure and produces more of the antibodies. This causes the release of chemicals in the body, which lead to an allergic reaction. Symptoms of an allergy can include sneezing, wheezing, itchy eyes, skin rashes and swelling. In very rare cases, an allergy can lead to anaphylactic shock, which in some extreme cases can be fatal. Most allergic reactions occur locally in a particular part of the body, such as the nose, eyes, or skin. In anaphylaxis, the allergic reaction usually happens within minutes of coming into contact with a particular allergen. If the patient has an allergy, which could cause anaphylaxis, the General Practitioner will prescribe an auto-injection kit of adrenaline to be administered in the event of anaphylaxis.

Patient's Issues and Objectives	Consultation Assessment and Plan	Signature	Date	Review Date
Allergies To relieve any associated symptoms of an allergic reaction, to avoid any recurrence	1. Discuss the allergy with the patient and, or relative and agree the plan of care.			
	2. Note the patient's and, or relative's understanding of the allergy, and any concerns or anxieties they have:			
	3. Note the past history of allergic reaction, how frequently it occurs, how often it has occurred in the last year and any treatments prescribed:			
	4. Detail what the patient is allergic to:			
	5. Highlight the symptoms experienced by the patient during an allergic reaction: | SNEEZING | BLOCKED, ITCHY OR RUNNING NOSE | RED EYES | STREAMING EYES | ASTHMA | WHEEZING | COUGH | | BREATHLESSNESS | HIVES | RAISED, ITCHY, RED, RASH | SWOLLEN LIPS | SWOLLEN TONGUE | SWOLLEN EYES | | SWOLLEN FACE | ABDOMINAL PAIN | VOMITING | DIARRHOEA | ATOPIC ECZEMA | SKIN DRY CRACKED AND RED |			
	6. Consult with the General Practitioner for advice regarding the severity of the allergy, and detail the advice given:			
	7. Note any specific instructions regarding the patient's allergy and the agreed plan of care:			

Copyright © 2020 Planning For Care Limited

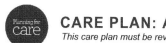

CARE PLAN: Allergy

This care plan must be reviewed monthly (or more often if required) and each action must be signed and dated

Patient's Issues and Objectives	Consultation Assessment and Plan	Signature	Date	Review Date
	8. Note any prescribed medication, and dosage, and how quickly it takes effect, where known:			
	9. Observe for any symptoms of anaphylactic shock which can include any of the following and administer the prescribed treatment: <ul><li>swelling of the throat and mouth</li><li>difficulty swallowing or speaking</li><li>difficulty breathing</li><li>a rash anywhere on the body</li><li>flushing and itching of the skin</li><li>stomach cramps, nausea and vomiting</li><li>a sudden feeling of weakness, due to a fall in blood pressure</li><li>collapsing and becoming unconscious</li></ul>			
	10. Liaise with General Practitioner as required.			
	....			

Name	Patient/Relative Signature	Date

Copyright © 2020 Planning For Care Limited

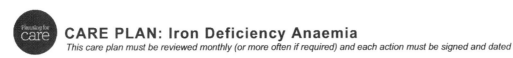

CARE PLAN: Iron Deficiency Anaemia

This care plan must be reviewed monthly (or more often if required) and each action must be signed and dated

Iron deficiency anaemia is a condition where a lack of iron in the body leads to a reduction in the number of red blood cells. The body needs iron, vitamin B12 and folic acid to produce more red blood cells. If there is a lack of one or more of these nutrients, anaemia will develop. Red blood cells take up oxygen in the lungs and carry it to all cells of the body. The cells use the oxygen to breakdown sugar and fat which then produces the body's energy.

Patient's Issues and Objectives	Consultation Assessment and Plan	Signature	Date	Review Date
Iron Deficiency Anaemia To maintain haemoglobin within normal levels To alleviate signs and symptoms of anaemia To prevent complications of anaemia To alleviate any concerns the patient may have	1. Discuss the condition with the patient and, or the relative and agree the plan of care.			
	2. Note the patient's and, or relative's understanding of the condition and any concerns or anxieties they have:			
	3. Note when the patient was first diagnosed, and any treatment they have received:			
	4. Highlight the cause of anaemia: | IRON DEFICIENT DIET | GASTROINTESTINAL BLOOD LOSS | INFLAMMATORY BOWEL DISEASE | COELIACS DISEASE | | MALABSORPTION | CHRONIC KIDNEY FAILURE |...........................			
	5. Highlight any of the following signs and symptoms experienced by the patient: | FEELING TIRED | LETHARGY, LACK OF ENERGY | LOOKING PALE | SHORTNESS OF BREATH | PALPITATIONS | | RAPID PULSE | DIZZINESS | HEADACHE | TINNITUS | DIFFICULTY SWALLOWING | ALTERED SENSE OF TASTE | | FEELING ITCHY | HAIR LOSS | BRITTLE SPOON SHAPED NAILS | SORES AT THE CORNER OF THE MOUTH | | SORE, SMOOTH TONGUE | DESIRE TO EAT ICE, PAPER, OR CLAY |.................................			
	6. Discuss the importance of eating foods rich in iron, highlight which iron rich foods the patient likes: | RED MEAT | EGG YOLKS | DRIED FRUITS | SHELL FISH | WHOLE WHEAT BREAD | CEREALS | RICE | POULTRY | | PEAS | BEANS | LENTILS | CHICKPEAS | DARK LEAFY GREENS | ARTICHOKES | LIVER |........................			
	7. Detail the agreed plan of care to assist the patient with any activities of daily living, that they have an issue with:			

Copyright © 2020 Planning For Care Limited

CARE PLAN: Iron Deficiency Anaemia

This care plan must be reviewed monthly (or more often if required) and each action must be signed and dated

Patient's Issues and Objectives	Consultation Assessment and Plan	Signature	Date	Review Date
	8. Note the name of the prescribed medication, dose and frequency:			
	9. The following are possible side effects of the prescribed medication, iron. Highlight any experienced by the patient: • black coloured stools • constipation • diarrhoea			
	10. Obtain bloods with the patient's consent and send to the laboratory for analysis annually, or at doctor's request.			
	11. Monitor the signs and symptoms of anaemia and liaise with the General Practitioner as required.			
	....			

Name	Patient/Relative Signature	Date

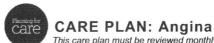

CARE PLAN: Angina

This care plan must be reviewed monthly (or more often if required) and each action must be signed and dated

Angina is a heart condition caused when the blood supply to the muscles of the heart is restricted. It usually occurs when the arteries which supply the heart become hardened and narrowed. The most common symptom of angina is a feeling of pain or discomfort in the chest. The pain can feel tight, dull or heavy and usually passes within a few minutes. The pain can spread to the left arm, neck, jaw and back. It usually follows a period of physical activity or emotional stress. In some cases, the pain can also develop after eating a meal or during cold weather. Some people with angina may also experience symptoms of breathlessness, nausea, fatigue, dizziness, belching or restlessness. Angina sufferers are at increased risk of developing a heart attack or a stroke and must be closely observed.

Patient's Issues and Objectives	Consultation Assessment and Plan	Signature	Date	Review Date
Angina To promote effective management of the condition To maintain an optimal level of independence and lifestyle	1. Discuss the condition with the patient and, or relative and agree the plan of care.			
	2. Note the patient's and, or relative's understanding of the condition and any concerns or anxieties they have:			
	3. Note the past history of angina:			
	4. Note any triggers which can cause the patient to have an angina attack: | NONE KNOWN | PHYSICAL ACTIVITY | EMOTIONAL STRESS | EATING A MEAL | COLD WEATHER |............			
	5. Highlight the symptoms the patient experiences during an angina attack: | HEAVY CHEST PAIN | TIGHT CHEST PAIN | | DULL CHEST PAIN | BREATHLESSNESS | NAUSEA | DIZZINESS | RESTLESSNESS | FEELING UNUSUALLY TIRED |			
	6. Highlight any contributing factors: | OBESITY | SMOKING | DIABETES TYPE I | DIABETES TYPE 2 | KIDNEY DISEASE | EXCESSIVE SALT | LACK OF EXERCISE | | EXCESSIVE ALCOHOL | MEDICATION, STEROIDS |...			
	7. Note any agreed plan for lifestyle changes where appropriate:			
	8. Note the agreed plan to avoid, or minimise the triggers which cause the angina attacks:			

Copyright © 2020 Planning For Care Limited

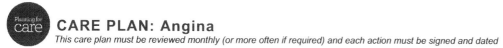

CARE PLAN: Angina

This care plan must be reviewed monthly (or more often if required) and each action must be signed and dated

Patient's Issues and Objectives	Consultation Assessment and Plan	Signature	Date	Review Date
	9. Note the prescribed medication, dose and frequency:			
	10. Note the patient's baseline blood pressure and pulse and note the frequency of monitoring:			
	11. Observe for any signs or symptoms of a heart attack, or stroke which can be a complication of angina, if present seek medical assistance immediately: • crushing central chest pain, pain in chest and left arm, neck and jaw • pain lasting for more than a few minutes • anxiety, nausea, vomiting • shortness of breath • abnormal heart rate • severe headache, weakness of the face, arm or leg • difficulty speaking			
	12. Liaise with the General Practitioner as required.			

Name	Patient/Relative Signature	Date

Copyright © 2020 Planning For Care Limited

CARE PLAN: Anticipatory or Advance Care

This care plan must be reviewed monthly (or more often if required) and each action must be signed and dated

The process of anticipatory or advance Care Planning ensures that the very important aspects of a patient's future care, and end of life care are discussed fully, with sensitivity. The wishes of the patient and their relatives can be explored and decisions can be made to ensure the patient's and relative's wishes are fully respected and met.

Patient's Issues and Objectives	Consultation Assessment and Plan	Signature	Date	Review Date
Anticipatory or Advance Care To assess the wishes of the patient and to anticipate future needs To achieve the best quality of future care and to comply with the wishes of the patient and, or the relatives.	1. Discuss with the patient and, or the relative, the need or wish of the patient for advance care planning, including their current physical and mental health and any specific illness or condition they have.			
	2. Note if the patient has a financial power of attorney, or guardianship, and the name address and telephone number of the person appointed:			
	3. Note if the patient has a welfare power of attorney, or guardianship, and the name address and telephone number of the person appointed:			
	4. Where the patient lacks capacity note the name of the General Practitioner, or psychogeriatrician who has assessed this and completed the required statutory certificate and date issued:			
	5. Note whether the patient has made a living will or advance decision regarding future medical treatment and care and detail the wishes expressed in it:			
	6. Discuss with the patient and, or relative, the patient's wishes for care should their condition deteriorate, including where they prefer to receive the care, and note in detail:			
	7. Detail the patient's, or relative's wishes for end of life care, including whether they want to be resuscitated:			

Copyright © 2020 Planning For Care Limited

CARE PLAN: Anticipatory or Advance Care

This care plan must be reviewed monthly (or more often if required) and each action must be signed and dated

Patient's Issues and Objectives	Consultation Assessment and Plan	Signature	Date	Review Date
	8. Record the patient's spiritual beliefs or values and the agreed end of life plan of care:			
	9. Note and have regard for the wishes of the patient's family:			
	10. Detail the patient's wishes or instructions regarding after death and funeral arrangements, particularly if they do not have family, or there might be differences of views between the family members healthcare: ……………………			

Name	Patient/Relative Signature	Date

CARE PLAN: Anxious, Agitated or Distressed Behaviour

This care plan must be reviewed monthly (or more often if required) and each action must be signed and dated

Anxious, agitated or distressed behaviour can be a manifestation of many different emotions, unease, frustration, boredom, fear, confusion, pain, a search for safety, or an inability to request help. For some patients there might be inappropriate verbal or motor activity. Anxious, agitated or distressed behaviour can include negative thinking, irrational thoughts and behaviour, hysterical behaviour, incoherent babbling, screaming or repetitive questions. Anxious, agitated or distressed physical behaviour can include walking back and forth, walking about, repetitive body motions, protective of particular things, or of his or her possessions, or shadowing another person.

Patient's Issues and Objectives	Consultation Assessment and Plan	Signature	Date	Review Date
Patient displays signs of having anxiety, agitation or distress **To develop an awareness of any specific causes** **To calm, comfort and alleviate anxiety, minimise agitation and minimise distress**	1. Discuss the issues with the patient and, or relative and agree the plan of care.			
	2. Describe in detail the way in which the patient presents himself, or herself, as being anxious, agitated or distressed:			
	3. Describe the circumstances physical, or psychological which may lead to the patient feeling anxious, agitated or distressed:			
	4. Highlight the trigger if known:	NOISY ENVIRONMENT	CROWDED ENVIRONMENT	CHANGE OF ENVIRONMENT		INCONTINENCE	CONSTIPATION	ROOM TEMPERATURE TOO WARM	URINE INFECTION	CHEST INFECTION		ROOM TEMPERATURE TOO COLD	....			
	5. Consider using and highlight any action which may assist in managing the patient's behavioural issue: • Attempt to diffuse the situation, change the immediate environment to accommodate the patient's wishes, appear calm, and speak slowly using clear and short sentences, avoid being patronising, avoid telling the patient to calm down, be courteous, use the patient's name. • Distract the patient with another task, situation or thought process instead of dwelling on the patient's issue. • Use art, music or other activities to help engage the patient and divert their attention away from the anxiety. • Do not argue or reason with a patient who has lost the ability to do so, and do not be confrontational. • Follow the patients thought pattern and try to enter the patient's sense of reality • If essential the use of white lies or validating the patient's beliefs can assist in managing or calming the situation Specify:			

Copyright © 2020 Planning For Care Limited

CARE PLAN: Anxious, Agitated or Distressed Behaviour

This care plan must be reviewed monthly (or more often if required) and each action must be signed and dated

Patient's Issues and Objectives	Consultation Assessment and Plan	Signature	Date	Review Date
	6. Specify where possible the agreed plan to comfort, reassure or calm the patient, note any phrases which may help:			
	7. Note prescribed medication if any, such as anxiolytics, antipsychotic, hypnotics, pain killers, tranquillisers, laxatives etc and record the dosage:			
	8. If necessary give and record the prescribed PRN, Pro Re Nata, medication as required, following the Care Home's protocol. Monitor the effects and any side effect of the medication.			
	9. Liaise with the patient's General Practitioner and/or the Psychogeriatrician as appropriate.			

Name	Patient/Relative Signature	Date

Copyright © 2020 Planning For Care Limited

CARE PLAN: Angry or Aggressive Behaviour

This care plan must be reviewed monthly (or more often if required) and each action must be signed and dated

Angry or aggressive behaviour can be a manifestation of many different emotions, frustration, boredom, fear, confusion, pain, search for safety, or inability to request help. It may include inappropriate verbal or motor activity. Angry or aggressive verbal behaviour can include shouting, swearing, or using foul and abusive language. Angry or aggressive physical behaviour can include hitting or scratching or attempting to do these things.

Patient's Issues and Objectives	Consultation Assessment and Plan	Signature	Date	Review Date
Patient displays signs of anger or aggression **To develop an awareness of any specific causes** **To minimise frustration, anger, aggression, reduce anxieties, calm the patient, promote a safe environment**	1. Discuss the issues with the patient and, or relative and agree the plan of care.			
	2. Describe in detail the way in which the patient presents him, or herself as being angry or aggressive:			
	3. Highlight any physical or psychological trigger which can result in the patient being angry or aggressive if known: | CHANGE OF ENVIRONMENT | NOISY ENVIRONMENT | CROWDED ENVIRONMENT | TEMPERATURE TOO WARM | | TEMPERATURE TOO COLD | CHEST INFECTION | URINE INFECTION | INCONTINENCE | CONSTIPATION | OTHER..			
	4. Consider using and highlight any of the following interventions that will assist: • Attempt to diffuse the situation, change the environment to accommodate the patient's wishes, appear calm, be courteous, use the patient's name, and speak slowly using clear and short sentences, avoid being patronising, avoid telling the patient to calm down. • Follow the patient's thought pattern, and try and enter their sense of reality. • Distract the patient with another task, situation or thought process, instead of dwelling on the patient's issue. • Maintain an adequate and safe distance from the patient. This should be more than the normal social distance, as when dealing with an angry, frustrated or aggressive patient, closeness may be interpreted as a threat. If necessary, walk away from the patient. • Stand at an angle to the patient to avoid appearing confrontational. Do not point and do not touch the patient. • Maintain normal eye contact, staring can be considered to be threatening, and avoiding eye contact can seem that you are being dismissive. Be aware of your reaction to the patient's behaviour and try not to show fear or anger. • Do not argue or reason with a patient who has lost the ability to do so, and do not be confrontational. • Use art, music or other activities to help engage the patient and divert their attention. • If essential the use of white lies or validating the patient's beliefs can assist in managing or calming the situation. Specify:			

Copyright © 2020 Planning For Care Limited

CARE PLAN: Angry or Aggressive Behaviour

This care plan must be reviewed monthly (or more often if required) and each action must be signed and dated

Patient's Issues and Objectives	Consultation Assessment and Plan	Signature	Date	Review Date
	5. Specify where possible the agreed plan to lessen frustration, anger or aggression:			
	6. Note the prescribed medication, if any, such as antipsychotic, anxiolytics, antipsychotic, hypnotics, pain killers, tranquillisers, laxatives and the dosage:..			
	7. If necessary, administer and record the prescribed PRN, Pro Re Nata, medication as required, following the Care Home's protocol. Monitor the effects and any side effect of the medication.			
	8. Liaise with the patient's General Practitioner and, or the Psychogeriatrician as appropriate.			

Name	Patient/Relative Signature	Date

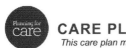

CARE PLAN: Bipolar Disorder
This care plan must be reviewed monthly (or more often if required) and each action must be signed and dated

Bipolar disorder, sometimes called manic-depressive disorder, is associated with mood swings that range from the lows of depression to the highs of mania. The exact symptoms of bipolar disorder vary from person to person. For some, depression causes most problems, for others, manic symptoms are the main concern. Symptoms of depression and symptoms of mania or hypomania may also occur together. This is known as a mixed episode. Mood shifts may occur only a few times a year, or as often as several times a day. Although bipolar disorder is a disruptive, long-term condition, it can be managed by following a treatment plan. In most cases, bipolar disorder can be controlled with medications such as mood stabilisers and antidepressants and psychological counselling.

Patient's Issues and Objectives	Consultation Assessment and Plan	Signature	Date	Review Date
Bipolar Disorder Mood swings from depression to mania To support the patient and manage the patient's mood swings to maximise their general well-being	1. Discuss the condition with the patient and, or relative and agree the plan of care.			
	2. Note the patient's and, or relative's understanding of the condition and any concerns or anxieties they have:			
	3. Note the medical history of bipolar disorder, how it affects the patient and any treatment previously prescribed:			
	4. Highlight any of the following signs and symptoms of depression experienced by the patient: | SADNESS | UNABLE TO GAIN PLEASURE FROM LIFE | LOSING INTEREST | HAVING NO ENERGY | POOR APPETITE | | INCREASED APPETITE | DIFFICULTY SLEEPING | WAKING EARLY IN THE MORNING | POOR CONCENTRATION | | FEELING RESTLESS | TENSE AND ANXIOUS | FEELING IRRITABLE | AVOIDING OTHERS | SUICIDAL THOUGHTS | | FINDING IT HARD TO MAKE DECISIONS| LACK OF CONFIDENCE | FEELING USELESS |...			
	5. Highlight any of the following signs and symptoms of mania experienced by the patient: | INFLATED SELF-ESTEEM | | EUPHORIA | | POOR JUDGEMENT | RAPID SPEECH | RACING THOUGHTS | DELUSIONS | EASILY DISTRACTED | | FEELING RESTLESS | AGGRESSIVE BEHAVIOUR | FEELING AGITATED | FEELING IRRITABLE | RISKY BEHAVIOUR | | INCREASED PHYSICAL ACTIVITY | DECREASED NEED TO SLEEP |...			
	6. Note anything which can trigger the patient's depression or mania:			
	7. Note the pattern of depression and mania experienced by the patient, and how it manifests:			

Copyright © 2020 Planning For Care Limited

CARE PLAN: Bipolar Disorder

This care plan must be reviewed monthly (or more often if required) and each action must be signed and dated

Patient's Issues and Objectives	Consultation Assessment and Plan	Signature	Date	Review Date
	8. Encourage the patient to express his or her feelings and thoughts and listen attentively.			
	9. Note anything which may improve the patient's mood:			
	10. Note anything which may calm the patient:			
	11. Identify any issues the patient has with safety and the agreed plan to address them:			
	12. Note and record the prescribed medication, dose and frequency if applicable:			
	13. Monitor the patient's mood and liaise with the General Practitioner as required.			

Name	Patient/Relative Signature	Date

Copyright © 2020 Planning For Care Limited

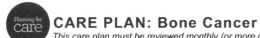

CARE PLAN: Bone Cancer

This care plan must be reviewed monthly (or more often if required) and each action must be signed and dated

Primary bone cancer is a rare type of cancer that begins in the bones. Secondary cancer in the bone is the result of cancer cells spreading to the bone from a primary tumour somewhere else in the body. Sometimes only one area of bone is affected, but in other cases the cancer spreads to a number of areas of bone. Secondary cancers in the bone might also be called bone secondaries. Bone secondaries often develop in different bones in the body, and not all bone secondaries will cause symptoms or problems. Although any type of cancer can spread to the bone, but the most common types which do are cancers of the breast, prostate, lung, thyroid and kidney.

Patient's Issues and Objectives	Consultation Assessment and Plan	Signature	Date	Review Date
Bone Cancer To maintain an optimal level of independence and lifestyle	1. Discuss the condition with the patient and, or relative and agree the plan of care.			
	2. Note the patient's and, or relative's understanding of the cancer and any concerns or anxieties they have:			
	3. Highlight the diagnosed stage of the cancer, where known: • Stage 1 the cancer is low-grade and has not spread beyond the bone • Stage 2 the cancer has still not spread beyond the bone, but is a high-grade • Stage 3 the cancer has spread into other parts of the body, such as the lungs			
	4. Note the past history of cancer, whether it is primary or secondary and any treatments prescribed or received:			
	5. Highlight the symptoms experienced by the patient: | PERSISTENT BONE PAIN | TENDERNESS IN A BONE | | SWELLING AND REDNESS OVER A BONE | LUMP OVER A BONE | WEAKENED BONE | RAISED CALCIUM LEVELS | | FRACTURE | PRESSURE ON THE SPINAL CORD | FATIGUE | UNEXPLAINED WEIGHT LOSS |			
	6. Note the prescribed medication, dose and frequency if applicable:			
	7. Detail any of the activities of daily living the patient has issues with:			

Copyright © 2020 Planning For Care Limited

CARE PLAN: Bone Cancer

This care plan must be reviewed monthly (or more often if required) and each action must be signed and dated

Patient's Issues and Objectives	Consultation Assessment and Plan	Signature	Date	Review Date
	8. Note the agreed plan of care to address the issues the patient has with any of the activities of daily living:			
	9. Monitor the patient's condition and liaise with the General Practitioner or Consultant as required.			

Name	Patient/Relative Signature	Date

Copyright © 2020 Planning For Care Limited

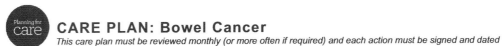

CARE PLAN: Bowel Cancer

This care plan must be reviewed monthly (or more often if required) and each action must be signed and dated

Bowel cancer is a general term for cancer that begins in the large bowel. Depending on where the cancer starts, bowel cancer is sometimes called colon or rectal cancer. Most cases of bowel cancer begin as small benign or non-cancerous clumps of cells called adenomatous polyps. Over time some of these polyps become bowel cancer. The main symptoms of bowel cancer are persistent blood in the stools, a persistent change in bowel habit, a persistent lower abdominal pain, bloating or discomfort, loss of appetite and significant unintentional weight loss. The treatment for bowel cancer may be a combination of surgery, chemotherapy and radiotherapy.

Patient's Issues and Objectives	Consultation Assessment and Plan	Signature	Date	Review Date
Bowel Cancer To promote effective management of the cancer To maintain an optimal level of independence and lifestyle	1. Discuss the condition with the patient and, or relative and agree the plan of care.			
	2. Note the patient's and, or relative's understanding of the condition and any concerns or anxieties they have:			
	3. Note the past medical history of bowel cancer, when it was diagnosed, and treatment received:			
	4. Highlight the symptoms experienced by the patient: | DIARRHOEA | CONSTIPATION | CHANGE IN CONSISTENCY OF STOOL | RECTAL BLEEDING | BLOOD IN STOOLS | | PERSISTENT ABDOMINAL PAIN | FLATULENCE | A FEELING THAT THE BOWEL DOES NOT COMPLETELY EMPTY | | WEIGHT LOSS | FATIGUE |..			
	5. Note all investigations carried out:			
	6. Highlight any contributing factors: | DIET HIGH IN RED OR PROCESSED MEATS | LOW FIBRE DIET | OBESITY | LACK OF EXERCISE | SMOKING | | EXCESSIVE ALCOHOL | FAMILY HISTORY |			
	7. Note any agreed plan for lifestyle changes where appropriate:			

Copyright © 2020 Planning For Care Limited

CARE PLAN: Bowel Cancer

This care plan must be reviewed monthly (or more often if required) and each action must be signed and dated

Patient's Issues and Objectives	Consultation Assessment and Plan	Signature	Date	Review Date
	8. Detail any issues the patient has with the activities of daily living, due to the condition, and the agreed plan to address them:			
	9. Liaise with the patient's General Practitioner as necessary.			

Name	Patient/Relative Signature	Date

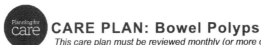

CARE PLAN: Bowel Polyps
This care plan must be reviewed monthly (or more often if required) and each action must be signed and dated

A bowel polyp is a small growth on the inner lining of the colon, large bowel, or rectum. Most bowel polyps are harmless, but over time some can develop into bowel cancer. They are common, and do not usually have symptoms. Polyps are usually less than 1cm in size, although they can grow to several centimetres. There are various forms, some are a tiny raised area or bulge, known as a sessile polyp, some look like a grape on a stalk, known as a pedunculated polyp, and some take the form of many tiny bumps clustered together. Some people just develop one polyp, while others may have a few. They tend to occur in people over the age of 60. Bowel polyps are caused by an abnormal production of cells. The lining of the bowel constantly renews itself, and a faulty gene can cause the cells in the bowel lining to grow more quickly. There may be a family tendency towards developing bowel polyps or bowel cancer. There are several methods for treating polyps, but the most common procedure involves snaring the polyp during a colonoscopy. Snaring is like cutting the polyp off with cheese wire and is painless.

Patient's Issues and Objectives	Consultation Assessment and Plan	Signature	Date	Review Date
Bowel Polyp To regain normal bowel function and promote effective management	1. Discuss the condition with the patient and, or relative and agree the plan of care.			
	2. Note the patient's and/or relative's understanding of the condition and any concerns or anxieties they have:			
	3. Note the past medical history of the bowel polyp or symptoms, when it was diagnosed, and treatments received:			
	4. Highlight the symptoms experienced by the patient: | NO SYMPTOMS | RECTAL BLEEDING | BLOOD IN STOOLS | BLACK STOOLS | MUCOUS IN STOOLS | DIARRHOEA | | CONSTIPATION | NAUSEA | ABDOMINAL PAIN | VOMITING | IRON DEFICIENCY ANAEMIA |............................			
	5. Detail any investigations which have been carried out:			
	6. Detail any planned treatment for the polyp, where applicable:			
	7. Detail any issues the patient has with the activities of daily living, due to the symptoms, and the agreed plan to address them:			

Copyright © 2020 Planning For Care Limited

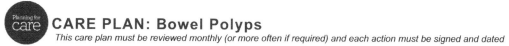

CARE PLAN: Bowel Polyps

This care plan must be reviewed monthly (or more often if required) and each action must be signed and dated

Patient's Issues and Objectives	Consultation Assessment and Plan	Signature	Date	Review Date

Name	Patient/Relative Signature	Date

CARE PLAN: Brain Haemorrhage

This care plan must be reviewed monthly (or more often if required) and each action must be signed and dated

A brain haemorrhage is bleeding in or around the area of the brain. The cause can include high blood pressure, abnormally weak blood vessels which leak, drug abuse, and trauma. Symptoms can include weakness on one side of the body, difficulty speaking, or a sense of numbness, and difficulty functioning, including problems with walking. In general, bleeding anywhere inside of the skull is called an intracranial haemorrhage. Bleeding within the brain itself is known as an intracerebral haemorrhage. Bleeding can also occur between the covering of the brain and the brain tissue itself, referred to as a subarachnoid haemorrhage. If a blood clot occurs between the skull and the brain, it is known as a subdural or epidural haematoma depending on whether it is below or above the dura of the brain. Subdural and epidural haematomas are more likely to occur as a result of a trauma or occur after a fall. When bleeding occurs within the brain itself, headache may not occur, as the brain does not have the ability to sense the ongoing disturbance. However, the coverings of the brain, called meninges, are extremely sensitive and if bleeding occurs there, a sudden and severe headache is a common symptom.

Patient's Issues and Objectives	Consultation Assessment and Plan	Signature	Date	Review Date
Brain Haemorrhage To maintain an optimal level of independence and lifestyle	1. Discuss the condition with the patient, and, or their relative and agree the plan of care.			
	2. Note the patient's and or relative's understanding of the condition and any concerns or anxieties they have:			
	3. Note the patient's past history, the type of haemorrhage, and treatment received:			
	4. Highlight any of the symptoms of stroke experienced by the patient: | SEVERE HEADACHE | SUDDEN CONFUSION | | UNABLE TO SMILE | WEAKNESS OF THE FACE | MOUTH HAS DROPPED | DIZZINESS | WEAKNESS OF AN ARM | | WEAKNESS OF A LEG | DIFFICULTY WALKING | LOSS OF VOLUNTARY MOVEMENTS | DIFFICULTY SPEAKING | | NUMBNESS |			
	5. Note how the haemorrhage has affected the patient emotionally, physically, and the areas of the body affected:			
	6. Note the agreed plan of care to address any issues the patient has with any of the activities of daily living:			

Copyright © 2020 Planning For Care Limited

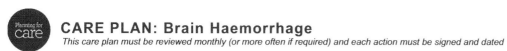

CARE PLAN: Brain Haemorrhage

This care plan must be reviewed monthly (or more often if required) and each action must be signed and dated

Patient's Issues and Objectives	Consultation Assessment and Plan	Signature	Date	Review Date
	7. Outline if the level of care required varies on a day to day basis and the reason:			
	8. Highlight any specialised equipment that may assist the patient: | ANTI SPILLAGE CUP | ADAPTED CUTLERY | NONSLIP TABLE MAT | PLATE GUARD | MECHANICAL HELPING HAND | | WALKING AID |			
	9. Note the prescribed medication, dose and frequency:			
	10. Liaise with the General Practitioner as necessary.			

Name	Patient/Relative Signature	Date

CARE PLAN: Brain Tumour

This care plan must be reviewed monthly (or more often if required) and each action must be signed and dated

A brain tumour is a mass or growth of abnormal cells in the brain or close to the brain. Many different types of brain tumours exist. Some brain tumours are noncancerous or benign, and some brain tumours are cancerous or malignant. Brain tumours which begin in the brain are primary brain tumours, and secondary, or metastatic, brain tumours cancer begin in other parts of the body and have spread to the brain. How quickly a brain tumour grows can vary greatly. The growth rate as well as location of a brain tumour determines how it will affect the function of your nervous system. Brain tumour treatment options depend on the type of brain tumour, as well as its size and location. Brain tumours damage the cells around them by causing inflammation and putting increased pressure on the tissue under and around it as well as inside the skull.

Patient's Issues and Objectives	Consultation Assessment and Plan	Signature	Date	Review Date
Brain Tumour To maintain an optimal level of independence and lifestyle	1. Discuss the condition with the patient, and, or their relative and agree the plan of care.			
	2. Note the patient's and or relative's understanding of the condition and any concerns or anxieties they have:			
	3. Note the patient's past history, the type of brain tumour, and the treatment received:			
	4. Highlight any symptoms experienced by the patient: | SEVERE PERSISTENT HEADACHES | SIEZURES OR FITS | | NAUSEA | VOMITING | BLURRED VISION | DOUBLE VISION | LOSS OF PERIPHERAL VISION | WEAKNESS OF AN ARM | | WEAKNESS OF A LEG | GRADUAL LOSS OF SENSATION | DIFFICULTY WITH BALANCE | DIFFICULTY WALKING | | DIFFICULTY SPEAKING | CONFUSION | PERSONALITY CHANGES | BEHAVIOURAL CHANGES | HEARING PROBLEMS | OTHER:			
	5. Note how the tumour has affected the patient emotionally, physically, and the areas of the body affected:			
	6. Note the agreed plan of care to address any issues the patient has with any of the activities of daily living:			

Copyright © 2020 Planning For Care Limited

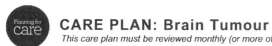

CARE PLAN: Brain Tumour

This care plan must be reviewed monthly (or more often if required) and each action must be signed and dated

Patient's Issues and Objectives	Consultation Assessment and Plan	Signature	Date	Review Date
	7. Outline if the level of care required varies on a day to day basis and the reason:			
	8. Highlight any specialised equipment that may assist the patient: | ANTI SPILLAGE CUP | ADAPTED CUTLERY | | NONSLIP TABLE MAT | PLATE GUARD | MECHANICAL HELPING HAND | WALKING AID |			
	9. Note the prescribed medication, dose and frequency:			
	10. Liaise with the General Practitioner as necessary.			

Name	Patient/Relative Signature	Date

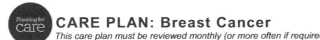

CARE PLAN: Breast Cancer

This care plan must be reviewed monthly (or more often if required) and each action must be signed and dated

Breast cancer starts when cells in the breast begin to grow out of control. These cells form a tumour which can often be seen on an X-ray or felt as a lump. If the cells grow into or invade surrounding tissues, or spread to distant areas of the body, the tumour is malignant. Breast cancer occurs mostly in women, but men can get breast cancer too. Often, there are no symptoms of breast cancer, but signs of breast cancer can include a breast lump or an abnormal mammogram. Breast cancer stages range from early curable breast cancer to metastatic breast cancer. There a variety of breast cancer treatments, such as surgery, radiotherapy, chemotherapy, hormone therapy and biological, targeted therapy. Breast cancer can affect a patient's daily life in different ways, depending on which stage of cancer they have and which treatment is administered.

Patient's Issues and Objectives	Consultation Assessment and Plan	Signature	Date	Review Date
Breast Cancer To maintain an optimal level of independence and lifestyle	1. Discuss the condition with the patient and, or relative and agree the plan of care.			
	2. Note the patient's and, or relative's understanding of the cancer and any concerns or anxieties they have:			
	3. Highlight the diagnosed grade of the breast cancer, where known: • Grade 1 or low grade, or well differentiated, in which the cancer cells look different from normal cells, and they grow in slow, well organised patterns, and not that many cells are dividing to make new cancer cells • Grade 2 or intermediate, or moderate grade, or moderately differentiated, in which the cancer cells do not look like normal cells and are growing and dividing a little faster than normal • Grade 3 or high grade, or poorly differentiated, in which the cells look very different from normal cells. They grow quickly in disorganised irregular patterns, with many dividing to make new cancer cells			
	4. Note the past history of breast cancer and any treatments prescribed or received:			
	5. Highlight the symptoms experienced by the patient: | BREAST LUMP | BREAST THICKENING | SWELLING IN ARMPIT | | LUMP IN ARMPIT | CHANGE IN BREAST SHAPE | CHANGE IN THE NIPPLE | CHANGES IN THE BREAST SKIN, DIMPLING | | RASH AROUND THE NIPPLE | BLOOD STAINED DISCHARGE FROM NIPPLES | NEWLY INVERTED NIPPLE |			
	6. Note the prescribed medication, dose and frequency if applicable:			
	7. Detail any of the activities of daily living the patient has issues with:			

Copyright © 2020 Planning For Care Limited

CARE PLAN: Breast Cancer

This care plan must be reviewed monthly (or more often if required) and each action must be signed and dated

Patient's Issues and Objectives	Consultation Assessment and Plan	Signature	Date	Review Date
	8. Note the agreed plan of care to address the issues the patient has with any of the activities of daily living:			
	9. Monitor the patient's condition and liaise with the General Practitioner or Consultant as required.			

Name	Patient/Relative Signature	Date

Copyright © 2020 Planning For Care Limited

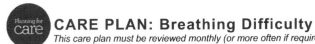

CARE PLAN: Breathing Difficulty

This care plan must be reviewed monthly (or more often if required) and each action must be signed and dated

Breathing difficulty or chronic obstructive airways disease, COAD, is the overall term used to describe a variety of illnesses, including chronic bronchitis and emphysema. People with COAD have permanently damaged lungs and find it difficult to breathe most of the time. Bronchitis is inflammation of the bronchial tubes that results in excessive secretions of mucous into the tubes causing the tissue to swell which in turn may narrow or close off bronchial tubes. Chronic bronchitis is defined as a cough that occurs every day with sputum production that lasts for at least 3 months, in two consecutive years. In emphysema, the air sacs are over inflated when air becomes trapped in them and their elastic fibres are destroyed. Small holes can develop in the walls of the sacs, leaving them unable to work properly.

Patient's Issues and Objectives	Consultation Assessment and Plan	Signature	Date	Review Date
Breathing difficulty To promote ease of breathing To maintain an optimal level of independence and lifestyle	1. Discuss the condition with the patient and, or relative and agree the plan of care.			
	2. Note the patient's and, or relative's understanding of the condition and any concerns or anxieties they have:			
	3. Specify the cause of the breathing difficulty where known:			
	4. Note the past history of respiratory issues and any treatments prescribed:			
	5. Note the frequency of acute breathlessness, whether, on exertion, or at rest, and any obvious specific trigger:			
	6. Note the prescribed medication, dose and frequency if applicable:			
	7. Detail the living conditions the patient prefers to help them psychologically or physically: Ventilation: .... Fans: .... Room temperature: .... Preferred position whilst in bed: .... Number of pillows required: .... Other relevant instructions:			

Copyright © 2020 Planning For Care Limited

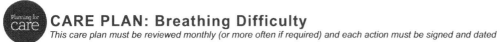

CARE PLAN: Breathing Difficulty

This care plan must be reviewed monthly (or more often if required) and each action must be signed and dated

Patient's Issues and Objectives	Consultation Assessment and Plan	Signature	Date	Review Date
	8. Highlight what the patient feels may help to relieve the acute symptoms: | GIVING REASSURANCE | STOPPING PHYSICAL ACTIVITY | HAVING AN OPEN WINDOW | SITTING UPRIGHT IN BED | | SITTING ON A CHAIR | STRETCHING ACROSS A TABLE | OTHER:			
	9. Ensure the patient has a sputum container or sufficient tissues for any expectorate, and monitor its appearance.			
	10. If sputum appears abnormal obtain a specimen and send to the laboratory for analysis. Note date sent:...			
	11. Ensure the patient has a buzzer at all times to enable them to summon help.			
	12. Monitor the patient's respiratory status, oxygen saturation levels and vital observations.			
	13. Monitor the patient's pallor and note any discolouration of extremities.			
	14. Monitor the patient's condition and liaise with the General Practitioner if required.			
	....			

Name	Patient/Relative Signature	Date

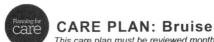

CARE PLAN: Bruise

This care plan must be reviewed monthly (or more often if required) and each action must be signed and dated

A bruise is a bluish or purple-coloured patch, which can appear on the skin when tiny blood vessels, called capillaries, break or burst. The blood from the capillaries leaks into the soft tissue under the skin, causing the discolouration. Over time, this fades through shades of yellow or green, usually around two weeks. Bruises often feel tender or swollen at first. A cold compress can be applied immediately, as it reduces the blood flow to the area and therefore limits bleeding into the skin and reduces the size of the bruise, it also decreases the inflammation in the area of the injury and limits swelling. If possible, the area should be elevated above the level of the heart. The lower an extremity is below the heart, the more blood will flow to the area and increase the bleeding and swelling. Bruising occurs more easily in the elderly because their capillaries are more fragile than those of young people. The amount of bruising may also be affected by medications such as ibuprofen, and aspirin, which interfere with blood clotting. Warfarin is often prescribed to prevent clotting in people who have had previous blood clots. It can cause severe bruising, especially if the level of the medication becomes too high. Cortisone medication, such as prednisone, can promote bruising by increasing the fragility of the tiny blood vessels in the skin.

Patient's Issues and Objectives	Consultation Assessment and Plan	Signature	Date	Review Date
Bruised Area(s) Promotion of healing and reduction of swelling	1. Discuss the bruise(s) with the patient and, or relative and agree the plan of care.			
	2. Note the cause of the bruising, and the patient's and, or relative's understanding of what happened and any concerns or anxieties they have:..			
	3. Apply a cold compress for 15-20 minutes every 1-2 hours to the bruised area. The manufacturers guidelines must be adhered to, as a cold compress can cause frostbite if applied directly to the skin or left on for too long.			
	4. Note where the bruise is on the patient's body and the dimensions:..			
	5. Consult the patient's General Practitioner for advice, and detail any advice:..			
	6. Note if there is anything which could be done to avoid any further risk of injury:..			
	7. Liaise with the patient's General Practitioner as required.			

Copyright © 2020 Planning For Care Limited

CARE PLAN: Bruise

This care plan must be reviewed monthly (or more often if required) and each action must be signed and dated

Patient's Issues and Objectives	Consultation Assessment and Plan	Signature	Date	Review Date

Name	Patient/Relative Signature	Date

Copyright © 2020 Planning For Care Limited

CARE PLAN: Bullous Pemphigoid

This care plan must be reviewed monthly (or more often if required) and each action must be signed and dated

Bullous Pemphigoid is an autoimmune disease, which causes the skin to blister. The blisters can be large, measuring up to 3cm across, and may be itchy and painful, they appear mainly on the trunk, arms, and legs. Occasionally, the inner lining tissue of the mouth, mucous membrane tissue, can be involved. This condition is not infectious. The majority of cases of Bullous Pemphigoid occur in people 50 years of age or older. The condition can resolve with topical cortisone creams but sometimes requires high doses of steroids taken internally. Severe Bullous Pemphigoid can also require immune-suppression drugs.

Patient's Issues and Objectives	Consultation Assessment and Plan	Signature	Date	Review Date
Bullous Pemphigoid To promote effective management of the condition To promote healing and maintain the integrity of the skin	1. Discuss the condition with the patient and, or relative and agree the plan of care.			
	2. Note the patient's and, or relative's understanding of the condition and any concerns or anxieties they have:			
	3. Note the patient's past history of the condition and treatment received:			
	4. Highlight any possible causes or triggers: • Non-steroidal anti-inflammatory drugs such as ibuprofen. • Drugs derived from penicillamine. • Herpes simplex virus. • Exposure to sunlight. • Long-term stress			
	5. Identify any area(s) affected with Bullous Pemphagoid:			
	6. Note any other symptoms the patient is experiencing:			
	7. Consult with the patient's General Practitioner.			

Copyright © 2020 Planning For Care Limited

CARE PLAN: Bullous Pemphigoid

This care plan must be reviewed monthly (or more often if required) and each action must be signed and dated

Patient's Issues and Objectives	Consultation Assessment and Plan	Signature	Date	Review Date
	8. Note the prescribed medication and treatment regime:			
	9. Identify any issues the patient has with the application of creams:			
	10. Identify any psychological issues the patient has due to the condition:			
	11. Liaise with the patient's General Practitioner as necessary.			

Name	Patient/Relative Signature	Date

Copyright © 2020 Planning For Care Limited

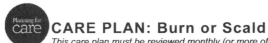

CARE PLAN: Burn or Scald

This care plan must be reviewed monthly (or more often if required) and each action must be signed and dated

Burns and scalds are damage to the skin caused by heat. Both are treated in the same way. A burn is caused by dry heat such as an iron, and a scald is caused by hot water or steam. Burns can be very painful and may cause red or peeling skin, blisters, swelling, white or charred skin. The amount of pain felt is not always related to how serious the burn is. Even a very serious burn may be relatively painless. For chemical burns, the chemical should be identified, and brushed off the skin if it is in a dry form, any affected clothing should be removed, and the burn should be irrigated with water for an hour. If the burn is caused by electricity, it should be switched off, or the person should be removed from the electrical source using a non-conductive material, such as a wooden stick, and immediate medical assistance must be sought.

Patient's Issues and Objectives	Consultation Assessment and Plan	Signature	Date	Review Date
Burn or scald To heal the Burn or scald and maintain the skin integrity	1. Discuss the issue with the patient and, or relative and agree the plan of care.			
	2. Specify the cause of the burn or scald:			
	3. Note the patient's and, or relative's understanding of the issue and any concerns or anxieties they have:			
	4. Where appropriate first aid treatment for a burn or a scald should be provided in the following manner: • immediately get the patient away from the heat source to stop the burning • cool the burn with cool or lukewarm running water for 20 minutes, do not use ice, or any creams • remove any clothing or jewellery that is near the burn, but don not move anything that is stuck to the skin • ensure the patient keeps warm • cover the burn by placing a layer of cling film over it • if the face or eyes are burnt, sit the patient up as much as possible, as this helps to reduce swelling			
	5. Highlight the type of burn or a scald the patient has: • superficial epidermal burn, where the epidermis is damaged, skin is red, slightly swollen and painful, but not blistered • superficial dermal burn, where the epidermis and part of the dermis is damaged, the skin is pale pink and painful, and there may be small blisters • deep dermal or partial thickness burn, where the epidermis and the dermis are damaged, the skin is red and blotchy, it may be dry or moist, and become swollen and blistered, and it may be very painful or painless • full thickness burn, where all three layers of skin, the epidermis, dermis and subcutis, are damaged, the skin is often burnt away, and the tissue underneath may appear pale or blackened, while the remaining skin will be dry and white, brown or black with no blisters, and the texture of the skin may also be leathery or waxy			
	6. Specify the location and area of the burn:			

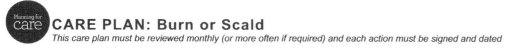

CARE PLAN: Burn or Scald

This care plan must be reviewed monthly (or more often if required) and each action must be signed and dated

Patient's Issues and Objectives	Consultation Assessment and Plan	Signature	Date	Review Date
	7. Consult with the patient's General Practitioner for advice and note the advice and prescribed treatment:			
	8. Note any prescribed treatment for pain management:			
	9. Complete a formal wound assessment chart, noting the size of wound, the type of wound, any exudate present, the depth of the wound and the condition of the surrounding skin, and review the wound as often as advised by the GP.			
	10. Note any assistance the patient requires with the activities of daily living and the agreed plan of care:			
	11. Monitor the wound and liaise with the General Practitioner and, or tissue viability nurse if necessary.			

Name	Patient/Relative Signature	Date

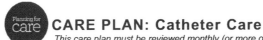

CARE PLAN: Catheter Care

This care plan must be reviewed monthly (or more often if required) and each action must be signed and dated

Urinary catheterisation is a medical procedure used to drain and collect urine from the bladder. A thin flexible tube is inserted into the body either through the urethra or through a hole in the abdomen. The catheter is then guided into the bladder, allowing urine to flow through it and into a drainage bag. A catheter may be prescribed to remove urine from the bladder if a person cannot control their bladder due to nerve damage or to treat urinary incontinence, loss of bladder control. It can also be used where there is incomplete emptying of the bladder, which if left untreated could lead to urinary tract infections or more seriously kidney damage. An intermittent catheter is where the catheter is temporarily inserted into the bladder and removed once the bladder is empty.

Patient's Issues and Objectives	Consultation Assessment and Plan	Signature	Date	Review Date
Catheterisation and Catheter Care	1. Discuss the prescribed procedure of catheterisation advised by the General Practitioner and gain the consent of the patient and, or relative.			
	2. Note the patient's and, or relative's understanding and any concerns or anxieties they have:			
To catheterise with privacy and dignity	3. Note the reason for catheterisation:			
	4. Highlight the type of catheter prescribed:	INTERMITTENT	INDWELLING CATHETER	SUPRA PUBIC CATHETER				
	5. Note whether the prescribed catheter is silicone or latex:			
To alleviate any anxieties	6. Note the batch number and expiry date of the catheter:			
	7. Note the catheter charriere (width) size:			
	8. Note the length of catheter:			
To maintain the catheter	9. Note the lot number and expiry date of lubricant used:			
	10. Note the planned date for renewal of the catheter:			
	11. Ensure the catheter is inserted by a trained person, using the correct aseptic technique.			
	12. Note the amount of sterile water inserted into the balloon (normally 10mls):			
	13. Note any issues with the insertion of the catheter, or post insertion:			
	14. Note any assistance required changing and emptying the catheter bag:			
	15. Ensure the patient's privacy and dignity are maintained at all times, when emptying, or attaching a drainage bag, also ensure the catheter and or catheter bag does not inhibit the patient's movement.			
	16. Ensure the patient's overnight catheter bag is changed each night.			
	17. Leg bags must be changed weekly, note the day for the change:			

Copyright © 2020 Planning For Care Limited

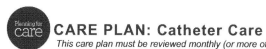

CARE PLAN: Catheter Care

This care plan must be reviewed monthly (or more often if required) and each action must be signed and dated

Patient's Issues and Objectives	Consultation Assessment and Plan	Signature	Date	Review Date
	18. Ensure the catheter bag is discreetly positioned and not visible to others, note where the patient prefers to have bag positioned during the day and night:			
	19. Observe for blockages within the catheter by monitoring urine output levels and any bypassing of urine.			
	20. Highlight the cause of any blockage: | TWISTED TUBING | ENCRUSTATION | CONSTIPATION | DETRUSOR SPASM |			
	21. Note any prescribed bladder management solution and the frequency:			
	22. Encourage the patient to have a fluid intake of 1500-2000mls per day for adequate hydration.			
	23. Note if there are issues with fluid intake and specify any assistance required:			
	24. Record in the patient's notes if there any issues with their urine or catheter.			
	25. Observe for any abnormalities in urine and if present obtain a urine specimen for multi stick analysis.			
	26. Consult the patient's General Practitioner if any abnormalities are observed in the urine and send a catheter specimen of urine to the laboratory for analysis.			
	27. Liaise with the General Practitioner regarding any issues with the catheter or the catheter care as required.			
	....			

Name	Patient/Relative Signature	Date

Copyright © 2020 Planning For Care Limited

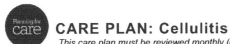

CARE PLAN: Cellulitis

This care plan must be reviewed monthly (or more often if required) and each action must be signed and dated

Cellulitis is an infection of the deeper layers of the skin and the underlying tissue. The affected area of skin turns red, and can be painful, swollen and hot. Cellulitis develops when the normally harmless bacteria, or fungus, move down through the skin's surface and into the underlying tissue through damaged or broken areas of skin, such as a cut, burn or bite. Skin conditions such as eczema or a fungal infection of the foot or toenails, athlete's foot, can cause small breaks and cracks to develop in the surface of the skin which can lead to a high risk of developing cellulitis. Complications of cellulitis can include the bacteria triggering a secondary infection somewhere else in the body such as the blood, septicaemia. Such cases usually require hospital admission for treatment with intravenous antibiotics.

Patient's Issues and Objectives	Consultation Assessment and Plan	Signature	Date	Review Date
Cellulitis To promote healing, to prevent recurrence and to relieve any associated pain	1. Discuss the condition with the patient and, or relative and agree the plan of care.			
	2. Note the patient's and, or relative's understanding of the condition and any concerns or anxieties they have:			
	3. Note the area of the patient's body affected by cellulitis and the dimensions of inflammation:			
	4. Assess and highlight which of the following symptoms apply: • signs of infection, skin red or inflamed • skin warm to touch • skin painful or tender to touch in the area with the rash or sore • areas of red skin increasing or spreading within the first 24 hours • areas of red skin with sharp borders or a tight glossy or stretched • appearance of the skin, hair loss at the site of the infection • stiffness of a joint caused by swelling of the tissue over the joint • nausea and vomiting • shivering and chills, feeling unwell Specify:..			
	5. Consult with the General practitioner for antibiotics, pain relief and, or other medication.			
	6. Note the prescribed medication and dosage:			

Copyright © 2020 Planning For Care Limited

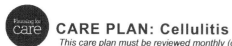

CARE PLAN: Cellulitis

This care plan must be reviewed monthly (or more often if required) and each action must be signed and dated

Patient's Issues and Objectives	Consultation Assessment and Plan	Signature	Date	Review Date
	7. Highlight the individual plan of care: • advise the patient to rest the area of body involved • encourage the patient to drink plenty of water • elevate the region of the body affected with cellulitis to decrease the main symptoms of swelling and to relieve irritation • if the area affected is the lower limbs use a bed cradle to alleviate pressure for bedding			
	8. Note in detail any additional agreed plan of care:			
	9. Complications of cellulitis include spread of the infection into the bloodstream or to other body tissues signs are: | RAPID SPREAD OF AREA OF REDNESS | FEVER TEMPERATURE OF 38C OR ABOVE | VOMITING | CONFUSION | | RAPID PULSE | RAPID BREATHING | DIZZINESS WHEN MOVING FROM LYING TO STANDING POSITION |			

Name	Patient/Relative Signature	Date

Copyright © 2020 Planning For Care Limited

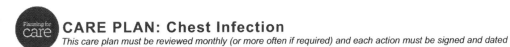

CARE PLAN: Chest Infection

This care plan must be reviewed monthly (or more often if required) and each action must be signed and dated

A chest infection is a bacterial or viral infection of the airways leading down into the lungs, or of the lungs themselves. The main types of chest infection are bronchitis and pneumonia. A virus usually causes bronchitis, whereas pneumonia is caused by a bacterial infection. Chest infections can range from being mild to life threatening.

Patient's Issues and Objectives	Consultation Assessment and Plan	Signature	Date	Review Date
Chest Infection To promote the healing process, to prevent recurrence, and to reassure the patient	1. Discuss the condition with the patient and, or relative and agree the plan of care.			
	2. Note the patient's and, or relative's understanding of the condition and any concerns or anxieties they have:			
	3. Record the patient's temperature, pulse, respirations, and blood pressure in the nursing notes.			
	4. If the patient has a productive cough, a sputum specimen should be sent to the laboratory for analysis. Date the specimen sent to the lab, where appropriate..			
	5. Consult with the General Practitioner, note advice and any prescribed antibiotics, cough mixture or other medication:			
	6. Highlight the agreed plan to ensure postural drainage, helping drain fluid from the lungs and helping breathing: • encourage the patient to sit up in a chair for periods throughout the day • encourage the patient to be in a upright sitting position when in bed			
	7. It is advised that the patient has 1500mls - 2000mls fluid intake per day, note any issues the patient has taking adequate fluids and the agreed plan to help the patient achieve this:...			
	8. Note any issues the patient has with the activities of daily living due to the chest infection, and the agreed plan to address them:			
	9. Monitor the patient's temperature, pulse, respirations, and blood pressure, daily or more frequently if required.			

Copyright © 2020 Planning For Care Limited

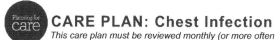

CARE PLAN: Chest Infection

This care plan must be reviewed monthly (or more often if required) and each action must be signed and dated

Patient's Issues and Objectives	Consultation Assessment and Plan	Signature	Date	Review Date
	10. Monitor the patient for breathing difficulties.			
	11. Liaise with the General Practitioner if there is no improvement by the 3rd or 4th day.			

Name	Patient/Relative Signature	Date

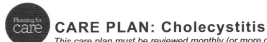

CARE PLAN: Cholecystitis

This care plan must be reviewed monthly (or more often if required) and each action must be signed and dated

Cholecystitis is inflammation of the gallbladder, a small organ on the right side of the abdomen beneath the liver. In most cases, gallstones blocking the tube leading out of the gallbladder cause cholecystitis. This results in bile build up which can cause inflammation. Other causes of cholecystitis include bile duct problems and tumours. Gallstones occur when bile, which is normally fluid, forms stones. Often just a few small stones are formed, but sometimes there are many. They do not usually cause symptoms, but they can occasionally cause episodes of pain, biliary colic, or acute cholecystitis. Acute cholecystitis is potentially serious and usually needs to be treated in hospital with rest, intravenous fluids and antibiotics. Possible life threatening complications are gangrene of the gallbladder tissue, or perforation of the gallbladder resulting in peritonitis.

Patient's Issues and Objectives	Consultation Assessment and Plan	Signature	Date	Review Date
Cholecystitis To effectively manage the condition To maintain an optimal level of independence and quality of life	1. Discuss the condition with the patient and, or relatives and agree plan of care.			
	2. Note any concerns or anxieties the patient and, or the relatives have:			
	3. Note any past history of gallstones or cholecystitis, including the tests that have been carried out:			
	4. Highlight which of the following symptoms the patient is experiencing: | SEVERE PAIN IN UPPER RIGHT SIDE OF ABDOMEN | PAIN RADIATING TO RIGHT SHOULDER OR BACK | | ABDOMINAL TENDERNESS | NAUSEA | VOMITING | HIGH TEMPERATURE | SWEATING | LOSS OF APPETITE | | JAUNDICE, OR YELLOWING OF THE SKIN | BULGE IN ABDOMEN |			
	5. Note any treatment received for the gallstones or cholecystitis:			
	6. Explain that eating a well-balanced, low in fat, low cholesterol diet is advised.			
	7. Note any instructions regarding the patient's diet and any issues they have due to likes, dislikes or memory issues:			
	8. Observe for any signs of complications, which can include the following, and seek immediate medical assistance: | ABDOMINAL PAIN | ABDOMINAL DISTENTION | FEELING OF FULLNESS | FEVER | LOSS OF APPETITE | NAUSEA | | VOMITING | DIARRHEOA | LOW URINE OUTPUT | THIRST | UNABLE TO PASS STOOLS OR GAS | FATIGUE |			
	9. Monitor the patient's condition and liaise with the General Practitioner or consultant as required.			

Copyright © 2020 Planning For Care Limited

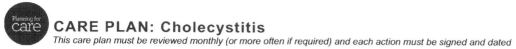

CARE PLAN: Cholecystitis

This care plan must be reviewed monthly (or more often if required) and each action must be signed and dated

Patient's Issues and Objectives	Consultation Assessment and Plan	Signature	Date	Review Date

Name	Patient/Relative Signature	Date

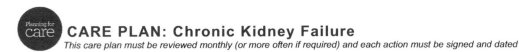

CARE PLAN: Chronic Kidney Failure

This care plan must be reviewed monthly (or more often if required) and each action must be signed and dated

The main role of the kidneys is to filter waste products from the blood before converting them into urine. The kidneys also help maintain blood pressure and the correct levels of chemicals in the body which, in turn, helps the heart and muscles function properly. The kidneys produce a type of vitamin D that keeps bones healthy and they produce a substance called erythropoietin, which helps stimulate production of red blood cells. Chronic kidney disease is the reduced ability of the kidney to carry out these functions in the long-term. This is most often caused by the strain placed on the kidneys by other conditions, most commonly diabetes and high blood pressure. There is no cure for chronic kidney disease, although treatment can slow or halt the progression of the disease and can prevent other serious conditions developing. People with CKD are known to have an increased risk of a stroke or heart attack because of changes that occur to the circulation.

Patient's Issues and Objectives	Consultation Assessment and Plan	Signature	Date	Review Date
Chronic Kidney Failure To promote the effective management of the condition To maintain an optimal level of independence and lifestyle	1. Discuss the condition with the patient and, or relatives and agree the plan of care.			
	2. Note any concerns or anxieties the patient and, or relatives have:			
	3. Note any history of previous kidney disease and the treatment received:			
	4. Note the cause of the kidney failure, where known:			
	5. Highlight which of the following signs and symptoms the patient is experiencing: | WEIGHT LOSS | POOR APPETITE | SWOLLEN ANKLES | SWOLLEN FEET | SWOLLEN HANDS | NAUSEA | FATIGUE | | HEADACHES | HYPERTENSION | SHORTNESS OF BREATH | INSOMNIA | PROTEIN IN URINE | BLOOD IN URINE | | INCREASED NEED TO URINATE, MORE AT NIGHT | DARK URINE | DECREASED URINARY OUTPUT | ITCHY SKIN | | MUSCLE CRAMPS |			
	6. Highlight the advice from the doctor regarding fluids or foods to be restricted: | FLUID RESTRICTION | SALT RESTRICTION | POTASSIUM RESTRICTION | SPECIFY:			
	7. Note the precise restrictions on fluids or specific foods:			
	8. Note any issues the patient may have with the restrictions:			

Copyright © 2020 Planning For Care Limited

CARE PLAN: Chronic Kidney Failure

This care plan must be reviewed monthly (or more often if required) and each action must be signed and dated

Patient's Issues and Objectives	Consultation Assessment and Plan	Signature	Date	Review Date
	9. Obtain a urine sample for multi stick urinalysis and note the result:			
	10. Note the arrangements with the renal unit for dialysis:			
	11. Note the prescribed medication, dose and frequency:			
	12. Monitor the signs of kidney failure, and observe for any signs of complications.			
	13. Liaise with the General Practitioner as necessary.			

Name	Patient/Relative Signature	Date

Copyright © 2020 Planning For Care Limited

CARE PLAN: Chronic Lymphocytic Leukaemia

This care plan must be reviewed monthly (or more often if required) and each action must be signed and dated

Leukaemia is cancer of the white blood cells. The stem cells, present in bone marrow start overproducing white blood cells, which are not fully developed. This overproduction of lymphocytes is at the expense of red blood cells, which are responsible for carrying oxygen around the body, and at the expense of platelets, which help stop bleeding. White blood cells help to fight infection, however, in leukaemia the immature white blood cells cannot fight infection. Symptoms can include repeated infections, tiredness due to a lack of red blood cells, bleeding and bruising, fever, night sweats, bone pain, weight loss, swollen spleen and swollen lymph nodes or glands. Some people can live for years or decades without developing symptoms or needing treatment. Treatment often involves chemotherapy, which cannot cure the condition, but can slow its progression and lead to remission. Regular blood tests help to monitor the condition. One of the main complications of chronic lymphocytic leukaemia is increased vulnerability to infection.

Patient's Issues and Objectives	Consultation Assessment and Plan	Signature	Date	Review Date
Chronic Lymphocytic Leukaemia To alleviate signs and symptoms To prevent complications of leukaemia To alleviate any concerns the patient may have	1. Discuss the condition with the patient and, or relative and agree the plan of care.			
	2. Note the patient's and, or relative's understanding of the condition and any concerns or anxieties they have:			
	3. Note when the patient was first diagnosed and any treatment they have received:			
	4. Highlight any of the following signs and symptoms experienced by the patient: | REPEATED INFECTIONS | FEELING TIRED | PERSISTENT TIREDNESS | LOOKING PALE | FEELING BREATHLESS | | DIZZINESS | RAPID PULSE | PALPITATIONS | BRUISING EASILY | FEVER | NIGHT SWEATS | SWOLLEN SPLEEN | | SWOLLEN LYMPH NODES | BONE PAIN | ABDOMINAL SWELLING | ABDOMINAL DISCOMFORT | WEIGHT LOSS |			
	5. Detail any issues the patient has with tiredness and how this affects their ability to carry out any activities of daily living:..			
	6. Detail the agreed plan of care and assistance the patient requires due to any of the symptoms they have:			

Copyright © 2020 Planning For Care Limited

CARE PLAN: Chronic Lymphocytic Leukaemia

This care plan must be reviewed monthly (or more often if required) and each action must be signed and dated

Patient's Issues and Objectives	Consultation Assessment and Plan	Signature	Date	Review Date
	7. Note the agreed plan of care to minimise the patient's risk of infection:			
	8. Note the prescribed medication, dose and frequency:			
	9. Monitor the signs and symptoms of leukaemia and liaise with the General Practitioner as required.			

Name	Patient/Relative Signature	Date

Copyright © 2020 Planning For Care Limited

CARE PLAN: Chronic Urinary Retention

This care plan must be reviewed monthly (or more often if required) and each action must be signed and dated

With chronic urinary retention, the patient may be able to urinate, but may have trouble starting or emptying their bladder completely. They may urinate frequently, or feel an urgent need to urinate but have little success when trying to, or they may feel they still have to urinate after finishing. With acute urinary retention, the patient cannot urinate at all, despite having a full bladder. Acute urinary retention is a medical emergency requiring prompt action. Chronic urinary retention can lead to serious problems and must also be treated. Men can experience urinary retention due to prostate enlargement. Women can experience this if their bladder sags or moves out of position, a condition called cystocele. The bladder can also be pulled out of position by a sagging of the lower part of the colon, a condition called rectocele. Urinary retention can also be due to nerve damage affecting bladder function. Urine is normally sterile, and the normal flow of urine usually prevents bacteria from growing in the urinary tract. When urine stays in the bladder, however, bacteria have a chance to grow and infect the urinary tract.

Patient's Issues and Objectives	Consultation Assessment and Plan	Signature	Date	Review Date
Chronic Urinary Retention To alleviate urinary retention	1. Discuss the condition with the patient and, or relative and agree the plan of care.			
	2. Note the patient's and, or relative's understanding of the condition and any concerns or anxieties they have:			
	3. Note the patient's past history of urinary retention:			
	4. Highlight the reason for the patient's urinary retention if known: | ENLARGED PROSTATE | DIABETES | MULTIPLE SCLEROSIS | PARKINSONS DISEASE | MEDICATION | SURGERY |			
	4. Highlight symptoms experienced by the patient: • difficulty in urinating despite adequate fluid intake • bladder distension • pain and discomfort in the region of the bladder and or kidney • frequent need to urinate, urinary hesitancy, urinary urgency, poor urinary stream, dribbling after passing urine, needing to pass urine throughout the night, new onset incontinence of urine throughout the night, a sensation of not emptying the bladder completely after passing urine • restlessness			
	6. Consult with the General Practitioner and highlight the treatment advised: • commence a fluid balance chart monitoring input and output of fluids • urinary catheter prescribed			

Copyright © 2020 Planning For Care Limited

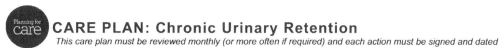

CARE PLAN: Chronic Urinary Retention

This care plan must be reviewed monthly (or more often if required) and each action must be signed and dated

Patient's Issues and Objectives	Consultation Assessment and Plan	Signature	Date	Review Date
	7. If a catheter is prescribed, note whether it is intermittent or indwelling or suprapubic:			
	8. If an indwelling catheter is prescribed note the catheter size, type and due date for replacement and ensure a catheter care plan has been completed:			
	9. Monitor effectiveness of treatment and liaise with the patient's General Practitioner as required.			

Name	Patient/Relative Signature	Date

Copyright © 2020 Planning For Care Limited

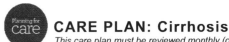

CARE PLAN: Cirrhosis

This care plan must be reviewed monthly (or more often if required) and each action must be signed and dated

Cirrhosis is scarring of the liver as a result of continuous, long-term liver damage. The scar tissue prevents the liver from working properly. The damage caused by cirrhosis can't be reversed and eventually can become so extensive the liver stops functioning. This is called liver failure. Cirrhosis can be fatal if the liver fails. However, it usually takes years for the condition to reach this stage and treatment can help slow its progression. There are many different causes of cirrhosis. The most common causes are drinking excessive amounts of alcohol and long-term hepatitis C infections. In some cases, no specific cause is identified. There are usually few symptoms in the early stages of cirrhosis. However, as the liver loses its ability to function properly, this can result in a loss of appetite, nausea and itchy skin. In the later stages, symptoms can include jaundice, yellowing of the skin and whites of the eyes, vomiting blood, dark, tarry-looking stools and a build-up of fluid in the legs, oedema and abdomen, ascites.

Patient's Issues and Objectives	Consultation Assessment and Plan	Signature	Date	Review Date
Cirrhosis To promote the effective management of the condition To maintain an optimal level of independence and lifestyle	1. Discuss the condition with the patient and, or relative and agree the plan of care.			
	2. Note the patient's and, or the relative's understanding of the condition and any concerns or anxieties they have:			
	3. Note the patient's past history of liver disease, the cause, any symptoms experienced, and any treatment received:			
	4. Highlight the cause if known: | ALCOHOL MISUSE | HEPATITIS C | HEPATITIS B | OTHER:			
	5. Highlight any symptoms experienced by the patient: | TIREDNESS | WEAKNESS | LOSS OF APPETITE | NAUSEA | | WEIGHT LOSS | VOMITING | MUSCLE WASTING | DROWSINESS | ITCHY SKIN | HAIR LOSS | FEVER | SHIVERING | | BLEEDING EASILY | BRUISING EASILY | TENDERNESS OR PAIN AROUND LIVER AREA | JAUNDICE YELLOWING SKIN | | YELLOWING OF THE WHITE OF THE EYES | TINY RED LINES ON THE SKIN ABOVE WAIST LEVEL | OEDEMA | | SWOLLEN LEGS | SWOLLEN ANKLES SWOLLEN FEET | SWOLLEN ABDOMEN ASCITES |..			
	6. Note the agreed plan of care to address any issues the patient has with any of the activities of daily living:			

Copyright © 2020 Planning For Care Limited

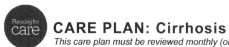

CARE PLAN: Cirrhosis

This care plan must be reviewed monthly (or more often if required) and each action must be signed and dated

Patient's Issues and Objectives	Consultation Assessment and Plan	Signature	Date	Review Date
	7. Consult the General practitioner for advice and detail any advice:			
	8. Note the prescribed medication, dose and frequency:			
	9. Observe for signs of complications and seek medical advice if the patient shows any of the following symptoms: • shortness of breath • vomiting blood • very dark or black tarry stools • periods of mental confusion or drowsiness			

Name	Patient/Relative Signature	Date

Copyright © 2020 Planning For Care Limited

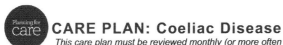

CARE PLAN: Coeliac Disease

This care plan must be reviewed monthly (or more often if required) and each action must be signed and dated

Coeliac disease is caused by a reaction to gluten, a protein found in wheat, and other similar proteins found in rye, barley and oats. When damaged and inflamed, the lining of the stomach is unable to absorb food properly, which often causes diarrhoea, malnutrition and anaemia. Other possible symptoms include mouth ulcers, vomiting and abdominal pain. There is no cure for coeliac disease, but following a gluten-free diet for life can control it. This allows the damaged stomach lining to recover and nutrients can then be absorbed normally again and symptoms can disappear. A diet rich in calcium and vitamin D and regular weight-bearing exercise are essential to help prevent osteoporosis from developing. Coeliac disease is more common among people with type 1 insulin-dependent diabetes, autoimmune thyroid disease, osteoporosis, ulcerative colitis and epilepsy. The condition runs in families. It is essential to consult a dietician to understand which foods are gluten-free fruit, vegetables, fresh meat, fish, cheese, eggs, and milk, and which foods contain wheat, barley and rye. The latter should be avoided or replaced with products such as rice or corn flour.

Patient's Issues and Objectives	Consultation Assessment and Plan	Signature	Date	Review Date
Coeliac Disease **To minimise pain and discomfort and to promote the effective management of the condition.** **To maintain an optimal level of independence and lifestyle**	1. Discuss the condition with the patient and, or relative and agree the plan of care.			
	2. Note the patient's and, or relative's understanding of the condition and any concerns or anxieties they have:			
	3. Note the past medical history of coeliac disease, when it was diagnosed, and any issues experienced:			
	4. Explain that a diet rich in calcium and vitamin D and regular weight-bearing exercise are essential to help prevent osteoporosis from developing. Agree with the patient and or relatives the gluten free diet plan.			
	5. Highlight the signs and symptoms the patient has experienced: | DIARRHOEA | BLOATING | FLATULENCE | ABDOMINAL PAIN | NUMBNESS | VOMITING | OEDEMA | WEIGHT LOSS | | MALNUTRITION | TINGLING | PERIPHERAL NEUROPATHY |..			
	5. Note any likes and dislikes with regards to a gluten free diet:			

Copyright © 2020 Planning For Care Limited

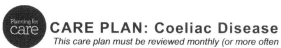

CARE PLAN: Coeliac Disease

This care plan must be reviewed monthly (or more often if required) and each action must be signed and dated

Patient's Issues and Objectives	Consultation Assessment and Plan	Signature	Date	Review Date
	6. Note any issues the patient may have with the diet and the agreed plan of care required to address them:			
	7. Monitor the patient's condition and consult with General Practitioner as required.			

Name	Patient/Relative Signature	Date

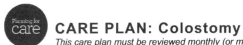

CARE PLAN: Colostomy

This care plan must be reviewed monthly (or more often if required) and each action must be signed and dated

A colostomy is a surgical procedure to divert one end of the large intestine, the colon, through an opening in the abdominal wall, the stomach. The end of the bowel is called a stoma. A pouch is placed over the stoma to collect waste products that usually pass through the colon and out of the body through the rectum and anus, back passage. This provides a new path for waste material and gas to leave the body. A colostomy can be permanent or temporary. When the colon, rectum, or anus is unable to function normally because of disease or injury, or needs to rest from normal function, the body must have another way to eliminate the waste. A colostomy may be used to treat the conditions such as, bowel cancer, Crohn's disease, Diverticulitis, Ulcerative colitis, and anal cancer.

Patient's Issues and Objectives	Consultation Assessment and Plan	Signature	Date	Review Date
Stoma care To effectively manage the colostomy and maintain skin integrity	1. Discuss the management of the colostomy with the patient and, or relative and agree the plan of care.			
	2. Note any concerns or anxieties the patient and or, the relatives have:			
	3. Note the past medical history and the reason the patient has a colostomy:			
	4. Specify the location of the patient's stoma:			
	5. Highlight any complications the patient has experienced as a result of the stoma: | SKIN IRRITATION | SKIN INFECTION | BLEEDING | CONSTIPATION | DIARRHOEA | BULGING AROUND THE STOMA | | SMELL | PSYCHOLOGICAL ISSUES | SPECIFY:.........			
	6. Discuss the importance of eating a well-balanced diet avoiding foods that cause excessive gas.			
	7. Note the prescribed colostomy products:			
	8. Note the agreed plan of care to manage the colostomy:			

Copyright © 2020 Planning For Care Limited

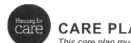

CARE PLAN: Colostomy

This care plan must be reviewed monthly (or more often if required) and each action must be signed and dated

Patient's Issues and Objectives	Consultation Assessment and Plan	Signature	Date	Review Date
	9. Monitor the regular function of the stoma.			
	10. Liaise with the General Practitioner and or stoma nurse if necessary.			

Name	Patient/Relative Signature	Date

CARE PLAN: Common Cold

This care plan must be reviewed monthly (or more often if required) and each action must be signed and dated

A cold is a mild viral infection of the nose, throat, sinuses and upper airways. It usually lasts for a week and usually causes a blocked nose followed by a running nose, sneezing, a sore throat and a cough. Taking over-the-counter medication, and drinking plenty of fluids can relieve the symptoms. Indications of spread of the infection to the chest, ears or sinuses are where the symptoms persist for more than three weeks, or where there is a high temperature of 39°C or above, or where blood stained phlegm is being coughed up, or there is chest pain, or breathing difficulties, or severe swelling of the lymph nodes, glands in the neck and or armpits. It is possible to have one cold after another, as a different virus causes each one. A cold can be spread through direct contact, through sneezing or coughing, where, the tiny cold virus droplets are breathed in. There can be indirect contact where the cold virus droplets are sneezed onto a hard surface such as a door handle, and then touched by another person. The contagious period is two to three days before the symptoms begin and continue until all the symptoms have gone. Most people will be contagious for around two weeks.

Patient's Issues and Objectives	Consultation Assessment and Plan	Signature	Date	Review Date
Common Cold **To promote the healing process, to prevent recurrence, and to reassure the patient**	1. Discuss the condition with the patient and, or relative and agree the plan of care.			
	2. Note the patient's and, or the relative's understanding of the condition and any concerns or anxieties they have:			
	3. Highlight the symptoms experienced by the patient: | BLOCKED NOSE | RUNNING NOSE | SNEEZING | HEADACHE | | COUGH | NASAL PAIN OR IRRITATION | EYE IRRITATION | HOARSE VOICE | MUSCLE PAIN | MILD TEMPERATURE | | FEELING UNWELL | LOSS OF TASTE | CONGESTION | EAR ACHE | FEELING PRESSURE IN EARS OR FACE | OTHER:..			
	4. Record the patient's temperature, pulse, respirations, and blood pressure in the nursing notes.			
	5. Consult with the General Practitioner for advice.			
	6. Note any prescribed medication and dosage:			
	7. Explain that the cold is contagious and stress the importance of good hand washing and infection control.			
	8. Note any assistance the patient may require to ensure the infection is not passed on to others:			
	9. Monitor the patient's temperature, pulse, respirations, and blood pressure, daily or more frequently if required.			
	10. Highlight the individual agreed plan of care: • encourage the patient to sit up in a chair for periods throughout the day • encourage the patient to be in a upright sitting position when in bed • encourage the patient to eat and drink adequate fluids			

Copyright © 2020 Planning For Care Limited

CARE PLAN: Common Cold

This care plan must be reviewed monthly (or more often if required) and each action must be signed and dated

Patient's Issues and Objectives	Consultation Assessment and Plan	Signature	Date	Review Date
	11. Note any additional agreed plan of care required for the safety, adequate hydration, postural drainage, comfort, and mental stimulation of the patient:			
	12. Monitor and observe the patient for any deterioration in their condition.			
	13. Consult the GP if the patient shows signs of the following as this can indicate the spread of the infection: • symptoms persist for more than three weeks • high temperature, fever, of 38°C or above • coughing up blood-stained phlegm, thick mucus • chest pain • breathing difficulties • severe swelling of the lymph nodes, glands, in the neck and, or armpits • confusion			

Name	Patient/Relative Signature	Date

Copyright © 2020 Planning For Care Limited

CARE PLAN: Communication Difficulty

This care plan must be reviewed monthly (or more often if required) and each action must be signed and dated

Communication difficulties can be particularly frustrating for elderly people and lead to feelings of depression and isolation. Nurses and carers should demonstrate patience and provide the patient with alternative methods of communication when possible, such as using lip reading, sign language, body language, or writing down what he, or she wants to say. Dementia is one of the major causes of communication difficulty, and can include difficulty in forming whole sentences, or recalling words or phrases. Other medical conditions, such as strokes and Parkinson's disease can also lead to communication difficulties, resulting in a total inability to communicate, or a decreased ability to communicate effectively. Poor hearing can also cause problems with communication. Patients with communication difficulties, which are related to dementia, strokes and Parkinson's disease, can also have comprehension difficulties which should be assessed as early as possible in order to maintain an optimum level of care.

Patient's Issues and Objectives	Consultation Assessment and Plan	Signature	Date	Review Date
Communication difficulty To promote optimal communication, and to improve understanding by both patients and staff	1. Discuss the communication issue with the patient and/or relative and agree the plan of care.			
	2. Note the patient's and or relative's understanding of the communication issues and any concerns or anxieties they have:			
	3. Highlight and detail the cause: | ALZHEIMER'S DISEASE | DEMENTIA | PARKINSONS DISEASE | VISUAL IMPAIRMENT | | STROKE | HEARING DIFFICULTIES | OTHER:...			
	4. Has the advice of an appropriate healthcare professional been sought and what advice or treatment was given:			
	5. Highlight and explain in detail how the patient communicates: | USES PARTS OF WORDS | GRUNTS | GROANS | VOCALISES | GESTURES | SIGNS | POINTS | MIMES | WORD BOARD | | USES A PICTURE BOARD | ALPHABET BOARD | USES SPEECH TECHNOLOGY | TOUCH SCREEN TECHNOLOGY | | DISPLAYS CERTAIN BEHAVIOURS OR ACTIONS | SPECIFY:...			
	6. Detail any issue the patient has with comprehension or understanding:			
	7. Consider using and highlight any of the following actions which may assist with communication: • on approaching the patient make eye contact and call the patient by his or her preferred name • ensure you are at the same physical level as the patient, and maintain eye contact • talk distinctly and clearly, facing the patient • repeat then rephrase if the patient appears not to understand • allow enough time for the patient to listen to what you are saying and to respond • observe for clues for an understanding by the patient of what was said • reassure the patient, encourage, and allow sufficient time for the patient to speak			

Copyright © 2020 Planning For Care Limited

CARE PLAN: Communication Difficulty

This care plan must be reviewed monthly (or more often if required) and each action must be signed and dated

Patient's Issues and Objectives	Consultation Assessment and Plan	Signature	Date	Review Date
	8. Specify the most successful way of interacting with the patient: .... **9. Specify any aids which would assist communication with the patient:**			

Name	Patient/Relative Signature	Date

CARE PLAN: Conjunctivitis

This care plan must be reviewed monthly (or more often if required) and each action must be signed and dated

Conjunctivitis, is a common condition which causes inflammation of the membranes, conjunctiva, covering the whites of the eyes and the membranes on the inner part of the eyelids. The conjunctiva can become inflamed as a result of a bacterial or viral infection, known as infective conjunctivitis, an allergic reaction to a substance such as pollen or dust mites, known as allergic conjunctivitis or the eye coming into contact with substances that can irritate the conjunctiva, such as chlorinated water or shampoo, or a loose eyelash rubbing against the eye, this is known as irritant conjunctivitis. Viral and bacterial forms of conjunctivitis are common in childhood, but they occur in adults as well. Other symptoms of conjunctivitis include itchiness and watering of the eyes, and sometimes a sticky coating on the eyelashes.

Patient's Issues and Objectives	Consultation Assessment and Plan	Signature	Date	Review Date
Conjunctivitis **To effectively treat the inflammation where possible and relieve any associated discomfort**	**1. Discuss the condition with the patient and, or relative and agree the plan of care.**			
	2. Note the patient's and, or the relative's understanding of the condition and any concerns or anxieties they have:			
	3. Note the patient's past history of conjunctivitis and the type if known:			
	**4. Which eye appears affected:	LEFT	RIGHT	BOTH	**			
	**5. Highlight the symptoms evident or experienced:	RED EYES	SORE EYES	GRITTY EYES	BURNING SENSATION		SEVERE PAIN IN EYES	WATERY EYES	BLURRED VISION	SWOLLEN LIDS	ITCHY EYES	RASH ON EYELIDS		PUS DISCHARGE	STICKY EYE LASHES	ENLARGED LYMPH NODE IN FRONT OF EAR	..........................**			
	6. Consult the General Practitioner for advice, detail the advice given, including the prescribed medication and dosage:			
	7. Discuss with the patient and, or the relative and note the agreed the plan of eye care:			
	8. Detail any issues the patient may have with the treatment and eye care and the agreed plan to address these:			
	9. Seek medical advice if the patient has signs of complications: • eye pain • sensitivity to light, photophobia • loss of vision • intense redness in one eye or both eyes			

Copyright © 2020 Planning For Care Limited

CARE PLAN: Conjunctivitis

This care plan must be reviewed monthly (or more often if required) and each action must be signed and dated

Patient's Issues and Objectives	Consultation Assessment and Plan	Signature	Date	Review Date

Name	Patient/Relative Signature	Date

Copyright © 2020 Planning For Care Limited

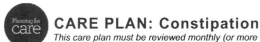

CARE PLAN: Constipation

This care plan must be reviewed monthly (or more often if required) and each action must be signed and dated

Constipation is medically defined as passing fewer than three stools per week and severe constipation as less than one stool per week. The causes of constipation can include, side effects of some medications, poor bowel habits, low fibre diets, abuse of laxatives, hormonal disorders, and diseases of other parts of the body that also affect the colon. Continually straining to pass stools can cause pain, discomfort and rectal bleeding. In some cases, bleeding is the result of a small tear around the anus, but, it can be caused by haemorrhoids, or piles. Chronic constipation can also increase the risk of faecal impaction, which is dried, hard stools collecting in the rectum and anus.

Patient's Issues and Objectives	Consultation Assessment and Plan	Signature	Date	Review Date
Constipation To regain normal bowel function and promote effective management	1. Discuss the condition with the patient and, or relative and agree the plan of care.			
	2. Note the patient's and, or relative's understanding of the condition and any concerns or anxieties they have:			
	3. Discuss and record the patient's normal bowel function, frequency, time of day and history of any bowel issues:			
	4. Highlight any contributing factors potentially causing constipation: | COGNITIVE IMPAIRMENT | CHANGE IN DIET | | IRON TABLETS | MEDICATION | POOR FLUID INTAKE | LACK OF EXERCISE | ANTIDEPRESSANTS | ANALGESIA |			
	5. Note any underlying cause for constipation, if known:			
	6. Note if the patient has the ability to complain of constipation and any agreed plan of care:			
	7. Highlight any signs and symptoms to suggest constipation, where the patient cannot express himself or herself: | AGITATION | AGGRESSION | PACING | INCREASED CONFUSION | RELUCTANT TO SIT | COMPLAINTS OF PAIN | | FACIAL EXPRESSION SHOWING DISCOMFORT | NAUSEA | RELUCTANT TO EAT OR DRINK | GUARDING ABDOMEN | | BLOATED |			
	8. Highlight the agreed plan of care that may assist in preventing constipation: • encourage adequate fibre intake 15-25g per day • encourage adequate fluid intake 1500-2000ml per day • encourage daily exercise • administer any prescribed medication as directed by the General Practitioner			

Copyright © 2020 Planning For Care Limited

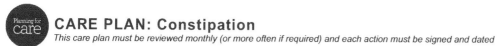

CARE PLAN: Constipation

This care plan must be reviewed monthly (or more often if required) and each action must be signed and dated

Patient's Issues and Objectives	Consultation Assessment and Plan	Signature	Date	Review Date
	9. Note any additional agreed plan of care:			
	10. Note if the patient has any issues drinking adequate fluids and specify any assistance required:			
	11. Note the prescribed medication, dosage and frequency:			
	12. Liaise with the patient's General Practitioner as required.			

Name	Patient/Relative Signature	Date

CARE PLAN: Covert Administration Of Medication
This care plan must be reviewed monthly (or more often if required) and each action must be signed and dated

Covert medication involves administering medicines in a disguised form, both in food and drink, to a patient who is refusing treatment, when this is necessary for the patient's physical or mental health and well being. The Mental Welfare Commission guidance makes it clear that a medical or other health professional must have assessed the patient and have issued a certificate of incapacity specifying that treatment in this manner that should be provided. The assessment should state that the treatment is necessary for the individual, and the benefit of giving covert medication must be sufficient to outweigh the risks of giving medication covertly. The assessment must take into account the risk that the individual may taste the medication in their food and drink, that this may damage their trust in staff, and that it may potentially lead them to refuse food or drink. Documented advice must be obtained from a pharmacist about how to administer the medicines covertly, before any administration takes place. Crushing or altering the original state of a tablet can be potentially dangerous. Any use of covert medication must be recorded, and the process of administration in this manner must be kept under regular review. If any additional medication is required, this must not be administered covertly but should be considered afresh and the decision on whether to administer this new medicine covertly must be justified in the same way.

Patient's Issues and Objectives	Consultation Assessment and Plan	Signature	Date	Review Date
Refusing treatment which is necessary for physical or mental health	1. Discuss with the patient and, or relatives about the issues the patient has taking their prescribed medication.			
	2. Note the patient and, or relatives understanding of the issues and any anxieties or concerns they may have:			
	3. Specify the reasons why the patient is refusing medication:			
To ensure the safe administration of covert medication	4. Note the benefits and risks to the patient, in considering whether covert medication should be introduced:			
	5. Note the patient's past wishes as to whether he or she is in favour of taking medication or treatment:			
To ensure the need to administer covert medication is reviewed regularly	6. Note if the patient has made a living will or advance decision regarding medical treatment and detail the wishes expressed in it:................			
	7. Name of the medical practitioner, psychogeriatrician who has assessed the patient and completed the Adults with Incapacity (AWI S47) certificate and the date:................			
	8. Note the reason the patient lacks capacity:			
	9. Note in detail any medicine which has been assessed and identified as necessary to be administered covertly:			

Copyright © 2020 Planning For Care Limited

CARE PLAN: Covert Administration Of Medication

This care plan must be reviewed monthly (or more often if required) and each action must be signed and dated

Patient's Issues and Objectives	Consultation Assessment and Plan	Signature	Date	Review Date
	10. Consult with the pharmacist and record any specific advice about giving the identified medications covertly:			
	11. Consult with the relatives and the pharmacist, note the agreed plan on how to disguise the medicine and the type and amount of food or fluids which is the safest and most acceptable:			
	12. Record in detail if the patient is unable to take or refuses to take the prescribed medication.			
	13. The patient should be assessed monthly or more frequently to review whether the covert administration of each identified medication continues to be necessary.			
	14. Liaise with the patient's General Practitioner or other healthcare professionals as necessary.			

Name	Patient/Relative Signature	Date

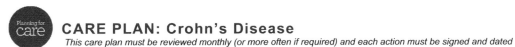

CARE PLAN: Crohn's Disease
This care plan must be reviewed monthly (or more often if required) and each action must be signed and dated

Crohn's disease is a chronic long term condition that causes inflammation of the lining of the digestive system. Inflammation can affect any part of the digestive system, from the mouth to the back passage, but most commonly occurs in the last section of the small intestine, or the large intestine. Crohn's disease can go into remission for long periods and be symptom free or have very mild symptoms. Remission can be followed by periods where symptoms flare up and become particularly troublesome. A complication associated with Crohn's disease is intestinal stricture where the inflammation of the bowel causes scar tissue to form, leading to the affected areas becoming narrowed causing a risk of bowel obstruction. Ulcers can also develop due to inflammation and over time they can develop fistula, a tunnel that runs from one part of the digestive system to another or, in some cases to the bladder, vaginal, anus or skin.

Patient's Issues and Objectives	Consultation Assessment and Plan	Signature	Date	Review Date
Crohn's Disease To regain normal bowel function and promote effective management of the condition	1. Discuss the condition with the patient and, or relative and agree the plan of care.			
	2. Note the patient's and, or relative's understanding of the condition and any concerns or anxieties they have:			
	3. Note the past medical history of Crohn's disease, when it was diagnosed, periods of remission and flare up, any treatment prescribed and how effective it was:			
	4. Highlight any signs and symptoms experienced by the patient: | RECURRENT DIARRHOEA | ABDOMINAL PAIN | | FATIGUE | BLOOD IN FAECES | MUCOUS IN FAECES | VOMITING | ARTHRITIS | NAUSEA | MOUTH ULCERS | FEVER | | INFLAMMATION AND IRRITATION OF THE EYES | AREAS OF PAINFUL, RED SWOLLEN SKIN | FEVER |............			
	5. Note the patient's normal bowel function: Frequency: Time of day:			
	6. Detail any issues the patient has with the activities of daily living due to the condition, and the agreed plan to address them:			
	7. Encourage sufficient fluid intake 1500mls- 2000mls per day, explaining the importance of this.			

Copyright © 2020 Planning For Care Limited

CARE PLAN: Crohn's Disease

This care plan must be reviewed monthly (or more often if required) and each action must be signed and dated

Patient's Issues and Objectives	Consultation Assessment and Plan	Signature	Date	Review Date
	8. Identify any issues the patient has regarding taking sufficient fluids and the agreed plan of care to address this:			
	9. Note the prescribed medication, dosage and frequency:			
	10. Observe for any of the following symptoms of bowel obstruction or fistula, and seek immediate medical assistance if present: • constipation, passing very watery stools • severe bloating • severe abdominal pain • vomiting • constant throbbing pain • high temperature, fever 38C or above • leakage of stools or mucous			
	11. Liaise with the General Practitioner as necessary.			

Name	Patient/Relative Signature	Date

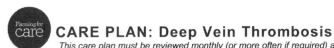

CARE PLAN: Deep Vein Thrombosis

This care plan must be reviewed monthly (or more often if required) and each action must be signed and dated

Deep Vein Thrombosis, DVT, refers to the formation of a thrombus or blood clot within a deep vein, commonly in the thigh or calf. The blood clot can either partially or completely block the flow of blood in the vein. A DVT can be caused by a narrowed or blocked vein, which allows the blood to clot. This can be brought on by an injury to the vein, such as a sharp blow to the leg, or following surgery or radiation therapy. It can also be caused by poor circulation as a result of inactivity or prolonged bed rest or as the result of severe infection, liver disease and some cancers. A DVT becomes life-threatening when a piece of the blood clot breaks off and travels downstream through the heart into the pulmonary circulation system, and becomes lodged in the lung. Diagnosis and treatment of a deep venous thrombus is meant to prevent a pulmonary embolism. The symptoms of a DVT may include pain, swelling, warmth and redness of the leg usually the calf. Various diagnostic tests can be used such as D-dimer blood test, ultrasound scan, a Doppler ultrasound or a venogram.

Patient's Issues and Objectives	Consultation Assessment and Plan	Signature	Date	Review Date
Deep Vein Thrombosis To manage the condition effectively	1. Discuss the condition with the patient and, or relative and agree the plan of care.			
	2. Note the patient's and, or relative's understanding of the condition and any concerns or anxieties they have:			
	3. Discuss with the patient and or relative any possible contributing factors and highlight them: | PREVIOUS VENOUS THROMBOEMBOLISM | FAMILY HISTORY OF THROMBOSIS | INACTIVITY AFTER SURGERY | | BED REST | OBESITY | HEART FAILURE | MEDICAL CONDITIONS SUCH AS CANCER |................			
	4. Highlight any symptoms which are evident: | PAIN | SWELLING | TENDERNESS IN LEG | ACHE IN AFFECTED AREA | | WARM SKIN AROUND AREA OF CLOT | SKIN RED |................			
	5. Identify the affected area and record the measurement of the circumference of the affected body part:			
	6. Note the type of diagnostic test carried out:			
	7. Note the prescribed medication and treatment regime:			
	8. Discuss the importance of having the patient's legs raised higher than their hips when resting. This helps to relieve the pressure in the veins of the calf and stops blood and fluid pooling in the calf itself and will help the returning blood flow from the calf.			

Copyright © 2020 Planning For Care Limited

CARE PLAN: Deep Vein Thrombosis

This care plan must be reviewed monthly (or more often if required) and each action must be signed and dated

Patient's Issues and Objectives	Consultation Assessment and Plan	Signature	Date	Review Date
	9. If warfarin is prescribed advise the patient to avoid taking any cranberry juice, cranberries, or products containing cranberries as it affects the warfarin therapy and ensure a warfarin care plan is completed.			
	10. Monitor for signs and symptoms of complications such as sudden or gradual breathlessness, or chest pain, or sudden collapse as this may indicate a pulmonary embolism which is a medical emergency.			
	11. Liaise with the patient's General Practitioner as required.			

Name	Patient/Relative Signature	Date

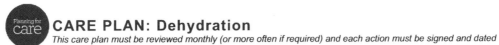

CARE PLAN: Dehydration

This care plan must be reviewed monthly (or more often if required) and each action must be signed and dated

Dehydration occurs when the amount of water leaving the body is greater than the amount being taken in. To test for dehydration, take the skin on the forearm or forehead using the index finger and thumb and squeeze gently. If the patient is dehydrated the skin takes time to return to its normal position.

Patient's Issues and Objectives	Consultation Assessment and Plan	Signature	Date	Review Date
Dehydration To maintain adequate hydration, and to maintain optimal health	1. Discuss the condition with the patient and, or relative and agree the plan of care.			
	2. Note the patient's and /or relative's understanding of the condition and any concerns or anxieties they have:			
	3. Discuss the importance of drinking adequate fluids with the patient and or relative.			
	4. Highlight the reason for the patient's dehydration: | MEMORY IMPAIRMENT NEEDS REMINDED TO DRINK | RELUCTANCE TO DRINK | SWALLOWING ISSUES | NAUSEA | | DIARRHOEA | VOMITING | EXCESSIVE PERSPIRATION | PHYSICAL DISABILITY | PARALYSIS |			
	5. Highlight the symptoms the patient is experiencing: | THIRSTY | LIGHTHEADED | DARK URINE | STRONG SMELLING URINE | PASSING LESS URINE THAN NORMAL | | DRY MOUTH | TIREDNESS |..			
	6. Record the fluid input and output on a fluid balance chart and assess how it may be improved.			
	7. Note the agreed plan of care required to assist the patient to achieve adequate hydration:			
	8. Note the patient's favourite drinks:			
	9. Monitor the patient's intake of fluids daily, 1500mls – 2000mls is a good fluid intake.			

Copyright © 2020 Planning For Care Limited

CARE PLAN: Dehydration

This care plan must be reviewed monthly (or more often if required) and each action must be signed and dated

Patient's Issues and Objectives	Consultation Assessment and Plan	Signature	Date	Review Date
	10. Refer to the General Practitioner if the patient's fluid intake is persistently inadequate.			

Name	Patient/Relative Signature	Date

Copyright © 2020 Planning For Care Limited

CARE PLAN: Dementia Alzheimer's Disease

This care plan must be reviewed monthly (or more often if required) and each action must be signed and dated

Alzheimer's is a disease where protein 'plaques' and 'tangles' develop in the structure of the brain, leading to the death of brain cells. There is also a shortage of some important chemicals in the brain, which are essential to the transmission of messages within the brain. It is a progressive disease, which means that gradually, over time, more areas of the brain may become damaged. In the early stages of Alzheimer's disease there may be lapses of memory and problems finding the right words. As the disease progresses, there may be increased confusion and forgetfulness. The person with Alzheimer's may experience mood swings, feel sad or angry, or scared and frustrated by their increasing memory loss. They may become more withdrawn, due either to a loss of confidence or to communication problems and have difficulty carrying out everyday activities. No two people are likely to experience Alzheimer's disease in the same way.

Patient's Issues and Objectives	Consultation Assessment and Plan	Signature	Date	Review Date
Dementia Alzheimer's Disease To maintain an optimal level of independence and quality of life	1. Discuss the condition with the patient and, or relative and agree the plan of care.			
	2. Note the patient's and, or relative's understanding of the condition and any concerns or anxieties they have:			
	3. Ensure the Life Story Book and a day in the life of the patient is completed and incorporated into this Care Plan.			
	4. Note when the patient was diagnosed and outline the past history of the condition:			
	5. Specify the type of issues or symptoms that the patient experiences:			
	6. Note any emotional or anxiety issues the patient has, how they are manifest, and the agreed plan to address these:			
	7. Assess the patient for pain, or showing signs of being in pain, record details, and the agreed plan to address this:			
	8. Assess the patient for depression, or showing signs of depression, record details and the agreed plan to address this:			
	9. Specify any issues the patient has with communication and the agreed plan to address these:			

Copyright © 2020 Planning For Care Limited

CARE PLAN: Dementia Alzheimer's Disease

This care plan must be reviewed monthly (or more often if required) and each action must be signed and dated

Patient's Issues and Objectives	Consultation Assessment and Plan	Signature	Date	Review Date
	10. Specify any issues the patient has with regards to safety, and any associated risks, and the agreed plan to address these:..................			
	11. Highlight any of the following activities the patient has issues with, or needs assistance with: | RISING FROM BED | GOING TO BED | USING WALKING AIDS | WALKING | MOBILISING | WASHING | DRESSING | | UNDRESSING | CUTTING FOOD UP | EATING | DRINKING | GOING TO THE TOILET | ATTENDING ACTIVITIES | OTHER..................			
	12. Note in detail what assistance the patient requires for the activities they have issues with:			
	13. Note the prescribed medication, the dose and frequency:			
	14. Liaise with the General Practitioner and/or Psychogeriatrician as required.			

Name	Patient/Relative Signature	Date

Copyright © 2020 Planning For Care Limited

CARE PLAN: Dementia Vascular

This care plan must be reviewed monthly (or more often if required) and each action must be signed and dated

Vascular dementia, sometimes called multi-infarct dementia, accounts for 20 per cent of all types of dementia. It is caused by small blood vessels in the brain becoming blocked which prevents oxygen reaching nearby brain cells, leading eventually to the death of those cells. It is likened to having many tiny strokes in the brain which cause a gradual decline in mental ability. This type of dementia is usually identified by sudden changes in behaviour. As more of the brain is damaged by these strokes, the dementia starts to resemble Alzheimer's disease. Vascular disease is treatable, and treatment may help to reduce the risk of further incidents to the brain. People with vascular dementia may experience problems with their speed of thinking, concentration and communication, depression and anxiety, physical weakness or paralysis, memory problems, seizures, or periods of severe, acute confusion. Other symptoms may include visual mistakes, changes in behaviour such as restlessness, difficulties with walking and unsteadiness, hallucinations, and delusions, problems with continence, and psychological issues such as becoming more obsessive.

Patient's Issues and Objectives	Consultation Assessment and Plan	Signature	Date	Review Date
Dementia Vascular To maintain an optimal level of independence and quality of life	1. Discuss the condition with the patient and, or relative and agree the plan of care.			
	2. Note the patient's and, or relative's understanding of the condition and any concerns or anxieties they have:			
	3. Ensure the Life Story Book and a day in the life of the patient is completed and incorporated into this Care Plan.			
	4. Note when the patient was diagnosed and outline the past history of dementia:			
	5. Specify the type of issues or symptoms that the patient experiences:			
	6. Note any emotional or anxiety issues the patient has, how they are manifest, and the agreed plan to address these:			
	7. Assess the patient for pain, or showing signs of being in pain, record details, and the agreed plan to address this:			
	8. Assess the patient for depression, or showing signs of depression, record details and the agreed plan to address this:			
	9. Specify any issues the patient has with communication and the agreed plan to address these:			

Copyright © 2020 Planning For Care Limited

CARE PLAN: Dementia Vascular

This care plan must be reviewed monthly (or more often if required) and each action must be signed and dated

Patient's Issues and Objectives	Consultation Assessment and Plan	Signature	Date	Review Date
	10. Specify any issues the patient has with regards to safety, and any associated risks, and the agreed plan to address these:..			
	11. Highlight any of the following activities the patient has issues with, or needs assistance with: | RISING FROM BED | GOING TO BED | USING WALKING AIDS | WALKING | MOBILISING | WASHING | DRESSING | | UNDRESSING | CUTTING FOOD UP | EATING | DRINKING | GOING TO THE TOILET | ATTENDING ACTIVITIES | OTHER............................			
	12. Note in detail what assistance the patient requires for the activities they have issues with:..			
	13. Note the prescribed medication, the dose and frequency:..			
	14. Liaise with the General Practitioner and/or Psychogeriatrician as required.			

Name	Patient/Relative Signature	Date

CARE PLAN: Dementia with Lewy Bodies

This care plan must be reviewed monthly (or more often if required) and each action must be signed and dated

Dementia with Lewy bodies may account for 10 to 15 percent of all cases of dementia in older people. Lewy bodies are tiny protein deposits found in nerve cells. Their presence in the brain interrupts the action of chemical messengers and disrupts its way of functioning normally. With similarities to Alzheimer's and Parkinson's, it causes impairment of memory, language and reasoning. It can also affect areas of the brain that control movement and balance as well as vision and recognition. People with Lewy body disease may have symptoms which include difficulty moving, which may result in falling and slowness, problems judging differences, hallucinations, agitation and disturbance. The person will experience many of the signs and symptoms of Alzheimer's disease and may also experience muscle stiffness, trembling of the limbs and a tendency to shuffle when walking. They may also experience hallucinations, seeing things that are not there, and fall asleep during the day and then not sleep at night.

Patient's Issues and Objectives	Consultation Assessment and Plan	Signature	Date	Review Date
Dementia with Lewy Bodies To maintain an optimal level of independence and quality of life	1. Discuss the condition with the patient and, or relative and agree the plan of care.			
	2. Note the patient's and or relative's understanding of the condition and any concerns or anxieties they have:			
	3. Ensure the Life Story Book and a day in the life of the patient is completed and incorporated into this Care Plan.			
	4. Note when the patient was diagnosed and outline the past history:			
	5. Specify the type of issues or symptoms that the patient experiences, particularly in relation to mobility, vision and speech:			
	6. Note any emotional or anxiety issues the patient has, how they are manifest, and the agreed plan to address these:			
	7. Assess the patient for pain, or showing signs of being in pain, record details, and the agreed plan to address this:			
	8. Assess the patient for depression, or showing signs of depression, record details and the agreed plan to address this:			
	9. Specify any issues the patient has with communication and the agreed plan to address these:			

CARE PLAN: Dementia with Lewy Bodies

This care plan must be reviewed monthly (or more often if required) and each action must be signed and dated

Patient's Issues and Objectives	Consultation Assessment and Plan	Signature	Date	Review Date
	10. Specify any issues the patient has with regards to safety, any associated risks and the agreed plan to address these:			
	11. Highlight any of the following activities the patient has issues with, or needs assistance with: | RISING FROM BED | GOING TO BED | USING WALKING AIDS | WALKING | MOBILISING | WASHING | DRESSING | | UNDRESSING | CUTTING FOOD UP | EATING | DRINKING | GOING TO THE TOILET | ATTENDING ACTIVITIES | OTHER:...			
	12. Note in detail what assistance the patient requires for the activities they have issues with:			
	13. Note the prescribed medication, the dose and frequency:			
	14. Liaise with the General Practitioner and/or Psychogeriatrician as required.			

Name	Patient/Relative Signature	Date

Copyright © 2020 Planning For Care Limited

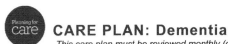

CARE PLAN: Dementia
This care plan must be reviewed monthly (or more often if required) and each action must be signed and dated

The term 'dementia' describes a set of symptoms which include loss of memory, mood changes, and problems with communication and reasoning. Alzheimers disease is the most common dementia. Damaged tissue builds up in the brain and forms deposits called 'plaques' and 'tangles', which cause the cells around them to die. It also affects chemicals in the brain, which transmit messages from one cell to another. In vascular dementia, the arteries supplying blood to the brain become blocked, this leads to small strokes when parts of the brain die as they are starved of oxygen. Lewy body dementia is caused by small protein deposits in the brain, and symptoms closely resemble Parkinson's disease. Fronto-temporal dementia is caused by damage to the front of the brain and is more likely to cause personality change. Huntington's disease causes dementia in younger people.

Patient's Issues and Objectives	Consultation Assessment and Plan	Signature	Date	Review Date
Dementia **To maintain an optimal level of independence and quality of life**	1. Discuss the condition with the patient and, or relative and agree the plan of care.			
	2. Note the patient's and, or relative's understanding of the condition and any concerns or anxieties they have:			
	3. Ensure the Life Story Book and a day in the life of the patient is completed and incorporated into this Care Plan.			
	4. Note the patient's past history of the condition if available:			
	5. Specify what type of dementia has been diagnosed or any memory issues experienced by the patient:			
	6. Assess the patient for pain, or showing signs of being in pain, record details, and the agreed plan to address this:			
	7. Assess the patient for depression, or showing signs of depression, record details and the agreed plan to address this:			
	8. Specify any issues the patient has with communication and the agreed plan to address these:			
	9. Specify any issues the patient has with regards to safety and any associated risks and the agreed plan to address these:			
	10. Highlight any of the following activities the patient has issues with, or needs assistance with: | RISING FROM BED | GOING TO BED | USING WALKING AIDS | WALKING | MOBILISING | WASHING | DRESSING | | UNDRESSING | CUTTING FOOD UP | EATING | DRINKING | GOING TO THE TOILET | ATTENDING ACTIVITIES |			

Copyright © 2020 Planning For Care Limited

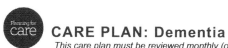

CARE PLAN: Dementia

This care plan must be reviewed monthly (or more often if required) and each action must be signed and dated

Patient's Issues and Objectives	Consultation Assessment and Plan	Signature	Date	Review Date
	11. Note in detail the agreed plan of care for the activities of living the patient has issues with:			
	12. Note any anxiety or emotional issues the patient has, how they are manifest and the agreed plan to address them :			
	13. Note the prescribed medication, the dose and frequency:			
	14. Liaise with the General Practitioner and, or Psychogeriatrician as required.			

Name	Patient/Relative Signature	Date

Copyright © 2020 Planning For Care Limited

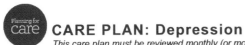

CARE PLAN: Depression

This care plan must be reviewed monthly (or more often if required) and each action must be signed and dated

A diagnosis of depression is made after assessing the severity of low mood, other associated symptoms and the duration of the problem. Unfortunately, there is no brain scan or blood test that can be used to diagnose when a person has a depressive illness. The diagnosis can only be made from an analysis of the symptoms.

Patient's Issues and Objectives	Consultation Assessment and Plan	Signature	Date	Review Date
Depression Recurring Low Mood To improve patient's low mood and to maximise general well-being	1. Discuss the condition with the patient and, or relative and agree the plan of care.			
	2. Note the patient's and, or relative's understanding of the condition and any concerns or anxieties they have:			
	3. Note any previous history of low mood or depression and any treatment previously prescribed:			
	4. Highlight any of the following signs and symptoms experienced by the patient: | UNABLE TO GAIN PLEASURE FROM LIFE | LOSING INTEREST IN LIFE | FEELING TIRED | HAVING NO ENERGY | | DIFFICULTY SLEEPING | WAKING EARLY IN THE MORNING | POOR APPETITE | INCREASED APPETITE | TENSE | | ANXIOUS | DIFFICULTY CONCENTRATING | FEELING RESTLESS | FEELING IRRITABLE | FEELING USELESS | | DIFFICULTY MAKING DECISIONS | LOSING SELF CONFIDENCE | AVOIDING OTHERS |			
	5. Encourage the patient to express his or her feelings and thoughts and listen attentively.			
	6. Identify any negative thinking patterns, or issues the patient has:			
	7. Discuss the benefits of exercise, good nutrition, good sleep pattern, social interaction and note any issues:			
	8. Note what action, if any, can be taken to help:			

Copyright © 2020 Planning For Care Limited

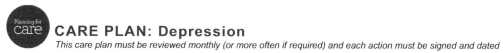

CARE PLAN: Depression

This care plan must be reviewed monthly (or more often if required) and each action must be signed and dated

Patient's Issues and Objectives	Consultation Assessment and Plan	Signature	Date	Review Date
	9. Note anything that may lift or improve the patient's mood:			
	10. Note and record the prescribed medication, dose and frequency if applicable:			
	11. Monitor the effects and any side effects of medication.			
	12. Monitor the patient's mood and liaise with the General Practitioner as required.			

Name	Patient/Relative Signature	Date

Copyright © 2020 Planning For Care Limited

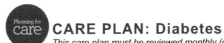

CARE PLAN: Diabetes

This care plan must be reviewed monthly (or more often if required) and each action must be signed and dated

Insulin is a hormone produced by the pancreas. It is needed to enable glucose, blood sugar, to move into the cells of the body, where it is stored and later used for energy. Type 1 diabetes occurs when the immune system destroys the beta cells in the pancreas that create insulin. As a result, the body makes very little or no insulin of its own. People with type 1 diabetes must be injected with insulin daily. Type 2 diabetes occurs when the pancreas does not make enough insulin or the body cannot properly use the insulin it does create. Complications that can occur are eye problems such as cataracts, diabetic retinopathy, glaucoma or foot and skin problems caused by nerve damage and blood vessel damage or heart problems.

Patient's Issues and Objectives	Consultation Assessment and Plan	Signature	Date	Review Date
Diabetes To maintain blood glucose level within the normal range, to understand and respect the patient's choices whilst supporting them to maintain optimal health	1. Discuss the condition with the patient and /or relative and agree the plan of care.			
	2. Plan the patient's diabetic diet in consultation with the patient and, or relative and the chef, explain the importance of careful management of the condition to avoid complications. Note any concerns they have:			
	3. Highlight which type of diabetes the patient has: • Type 2 diet controlled • Type 2 hypoglycaemic medicated and diet controlled • Type 1 prescribed insulin injections			
	4. Note the patient's past history of diabetes, when it was diagnosed, how stable the blood sugar levels are, note any issues:..			
	5. Highlight the symptoms the patient has experienced as a result of the diabetes: | FEELING THIRSTY | URINATING MORE FREQUENTLY | FATIGUE | WEIGHT LOSS | FREQUENT EPISODES OF THRUSH | | SLOW HEALING OF CUTS OR WOUNDS | BLURRED VISION |..			
	6. Note any instructions regarding the patient's diet and any issues they have due to likes, dislikes or memory issues:			
	7. Note the prescribed medication for diabetes, the frequency and dosage:			
	8. Note the General Practitioner's requirements regarding how frequently the patient's blood sugar levels and, or urinalysis should be checked:			

Copyright © 2020 Planning For Care Limited

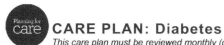

CARE PLAN: Diabetes
This care plan must be reviewed monthly (or more often if required) and each action must be signed and dated

Patient's Issues and Objectives	Consultation Assessment and Plan	Signature	Date	Review Date
	9. If the patient shows signs and symptoms of hypoglycaemia, low blood sugar, such as, trembling, shaking, sweating, fast pulse, palpitations, anxiety, irritability, hunger, tingling lips, their blood sugars and urinalysis should be checked.			
	10. If the blood sugar is low, encourage the patient to take a glucose drink.			
	11. If the patient shows signs and symptoms of hyperglycaemia, high blood sugar, such as increased thirst, fatigue, poor concentration, headaches blurred vision, frequent urinating, their urinalysis and blood sugar should be checked.			
	12. If the blood sugar is high and the urinalysis shows ketones the patient should be encouraged to drink water.			
	13. Ensure the patient has regular chiropody attention.			
	14. Ensure care is taken when manicuring or cutting the patient's fingernails.			
	15. Monitor the patient's skin integrity on an ongoing daily basis. Note if there are any issues:			
	16. Ensure an annual, or more frequent if required, examination is carried out by an optometrist.			
	17. Consult the Dietician or General Practitioner as required.			
	....			

Name	Patient/Relative Signature	Date

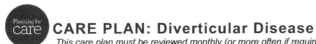

CARE PLAN: Diverticular Disease

This care plan must be reviewed monthly (or more often if required) and each action must be signed and dated

Diverticulosis is the formation of abnormal pouches, diverticula, in the bowel wall. Diverticulitis is inflammation or infection of these pouches. These conditions are known as diverticular disease. Diverticulosis is common and frequently has no symptoms, however, when many diverticula are present, the normal smooth working of the bowel can be affected. This may cause a range of symptoms including abdominal pain, bloating, constipation, diarrhoea, flatulence and blood in the faeces. This bleeding is usually minor, but can sometimes be heavy if a diverticulum gets inflamed or is near a blood vessel. Diverticulitis may be painful and disabling and can often be a medical emergency. Symptoms of diverticulitis may include a sharp pain, often located at a specific point, in the lower left half of the abdomen, fever, chills, distension, bloating of the abdomen, nausea and vomiting. Complications of diverticular disease may result in an abscess, hemorrhage, bowel obstruction, perforation of the bowel wall where the bowel contents seep into the abdominal cavity, or peritonitis infection of the membranes lining the abdominal cavity. A perforated bowel is a medical emergency.

Patient's Issues and Objectives	Consultation Assessment and Plan	Signature	Date	Review Date
Diverticular Disease To regain normal bowel function and promote effective management	1. Discuss the condition with the patient and, or relative and agree the plan of care.			
	2. Note the patient's and, or relative's understanding of the condition and any concerns or anxieties they have:			
	3. Note the past medical history of diverticular disease, when and how it was diagnosed, and any treatment prescribed:			
	4. Note the patient's normal bowel function and pattern: Frequency................................Time of day...................			
	5. Highlight any symptoms experienced by the patient: | ABDOMINAL PAIN | ABDOMINAL TENDERNESS | FEVER | | SEVERE OR SUDDEN ABDOMINAL PAIN LOWER LEFT SIDE | CHANGES IN BOWEL HABIT | CONSTIPATION | | DIARRHOEA | ABDOMINAL PAIN AFTER EATING | FEELING BLOATED | NAUSEA | VOMITTING | RECTAL BLEEDING |			
	6. Discuss with the patient and, or relatives the importance of eating a high fibre diet and note any issues the patient has eating a high fibre diet:			
	7. Detail any issues the patient has with any of the activities of daily living due to the condition and the agreed assistance required:			

Copyright © 2020 Planning For Care Limited

CARE PLAN: Diverticular Disease

This care plan must be reviewed monthly (or more often if required) and each action must be signed and dated

Patient's Issues and Objectives	Consultation Assessment and Plan	Signature	Date	Review Date
	8. Note the prescribed medication, dose and frequency:			
	9. Encourage sufficient fluid intake 1,500mls – 2,000mls per day.			
	10. Note if there are any issues with the patient drinking adequate fluids and note the agreed plan to improve this:			
	11. Observe for any of the following complications, and seek immediate medical assistance if suspected: • Heavy rectal bleeding • Bladder problems • Bowel obstruction • Fistula • Abscess • Peritonitis			
	....			

Name	Patient/Relative Signature	Date

CARE PLAN: Dressing and Undressing

This care plan must be reviewed monthly (or more often if required) and each action must be signed and dated

Dressing and spending time on personal grooming, in general makes people feel better about themselves by boosting confidence and self-esteem. It has a positive effect both physically and psychologically.

Patient's Issues and Objectives	Consultation Assessment and Plan	Signature	Date	Review Date
Dressing and undressing To ensure the patient's dressing and grooming is in accordance with the patient's choice	1. Discuss with the patient and, or relative any issues experienced by the patient, in relation to dressing and personal grooming and identify and agree where assistance would be beneficial.			
	2. Highlight what assistance the patient needs to choose their clothes: | INDEPENDENT | NEEDS ENCOURAGEMENT | | NEEDS HELP OR GUIDANCE | VARIES DAILY | ………………………………………………………			
	3. Highlight the items of clothing the patient needs assistance with dressing or undressing: | BRA | VEST | CORSET | GIRDLE | UNDERSKIRT | UNDER PANTS | INCONTINENCE WEAR | TIGHTS | STOCKINGS | | SOCKS | SKIRT | BLOUSE | CARDIGAN | SWEATER | DRESS | TROUSERS | T-SHIRT | SHIRT | TIE | BELT | BRACES | | JACKET | COAT | SHOES | LACES | ZIPS | BUTTONS | VARIES DAILY | …………………………………………………			
	4. Note any particular likes or dislikes the patient has: …… ……			
	5. Detail the agreed plan of care regarding dressing or grooming, and any specific requests: …… …… …… ……			
	6. Note if the level of assistance required varies from day to day and the reason why: ……			
	7. Highlight or note the patient's preferred environment for dressing or undressing: | BEDROOM | BATHROOM | VARIES DAILY | …………………………………………………………………			
	8. Note how frequently the patient requires to change clothes throughout the day and state the reason why: …… ……			
	9. Highlight the assistance required for care of the patient's hair: | SELF CARE | REMIND TO BRUSH HAIR | | ASSIST WITH BRUSHING HAIR | ………………………………………………………………………………… ……			

Copyright © 2020 Planning For Care Limited

CARE PLAN: Dressing and Undressing

This care plan must be reviewed monthly (or more often if required) and each action must be signed and dated

Patient's Issues and Objectives	Consultation Assessment and Plan	Signature	Date	Review Date
	10. Note how frequently the patient likes to get his, or her hair washed:			
	11. Note what makeup, if any, the patient prefers to put on and detail any assistance required:			
	12. Note any jewellery the patient likes to wear regularly:			
	13. Note if the patient has glasses or a hearing aid:			
	14. Note any specific requests made by the patient:			

Name	Patient/Relative Signature	Date

Copyright © 2020 Planning For Care Limited

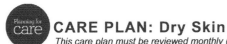

CARE PLAN: Dry Skin

This care plan must be reviewed monthly (or more often if required) and each action must be signed and dated

An elderly person tends to have diminished amounts of natural skin oils. When oils in the skin are stripped away or diminished, the skin loses its protection. Areas such as the arms, hands and lower legs tend to be more affected by dry skin. Symptoms include discomfort from skin tightness and itching. Cold or dry air and winter weather can worsen dry skin. As skin becomes dry it may also become more sensitive and prone to rashes and breakdown. If left untreated it may result in complications including eczema, secondary bacterial infection, cellulitis and skin discolouration. Fortunately, dry skin is usually mild and can be treated easily.

Patient's Issues and Objectives	Consultation Assessment and Plan	Signature	Date	Review Date
Dry Skin Promotion and maintenance of healthy skin	1. Discuss the condition with the patient and, or relative and agree the plan of care.			
	2. Note the patient's and, or relative's understanding of the condition and any concerns or anxieties they have:			
	3. Note any past history of dry skin conditions and treatments:			
	4. Highlight and discuss with the patient and/or the relatives any possible contributing factors: | COLD WEATHER | INFECTION | HARSH SOAPS | FREQUENT HOT BATHS | FREQUENT SHOWERS | SWEATING | | STRESS | ALLERGIES | POOR LOWER LIMB CIRCULATION | HEAT | OTHER:...................			
	5. Note the agreed plan of care to reduce or eliminate any contributing factors:			
	6. Identify the area/s affected by dry skin:			
	7. Consult with the patient's General Practitioner.			

Copyright © 2020 Planning For Care Limited

CARE PLAN: Dry Skin

This care plan must be reviewed monthly (or more often if required) and each action must be signed and dated

Patient's Issues and Objectives	Consultation Assessment and Plan	Signature	Date	Review Date
	8. Note the prescribed medication, dosage, and treatment regime:			
	9. Identify any issues the patient may have with the application of creams:			
	10. Monitor the effectiveness of the treatment and skin condition.			
	11. Liaise with the patient's General Practitioner as required.			

Name	Patient/Relative Signature	Date

Copyright © 2020 Planning For Care Limited

CARE PLAN: Ear Infection Outer Ear

This care plan must be reviewed monthly (or more often if required) and each action must be signed and dated

An ear infection is generally caused by a bacterial infection of the skin of the canal, although occasionally it may be due to a fungus or yeast. The skin can become so swollen that the ear canal closes, causing temporary deafness, and there can be a scanty discharge from the ear. It occurs commonly in people who suffer from skin problems such as eczema, psoriasis or dermatitis, but also in people with narrow ear canals or who swim a great deal. It can affect both ears and often keeps recurring, especially if a patient is rundown or stressed. Treatment for outer ear infections is generally in the form of antibiotic eardrops, which are instilled into the ear canal for at least a week. Sometimes antibiotics by mouth will also be necessary. In severe cases referral to an ear nose and throat specialist is both necessary and appropriate for cleaning of the ear canal and for more intensive treatment. An ear infection can be extremely painful with the result that sleep may be difficult.

Patient's Issues and Objectives	Consultation Assessment and Plan	Signature	Date	Review Date
Ear Infection To relieve any associated symptoms and effectively treat the infection	1. Discuss the presence of an ear infection with the patient and, or relative and agree the plan of care.			
	2. Note the patient's and, or relative's understanding of the issue and any concerns or anxieties they have:			
	3. Note the patient's past history of issues with ear infections:			
	4. Which ear is affected: | LEFT | RIGHT | BOTH |			
	5. Highlight the symptoms evident or experienced: | EAR ACHE | PAIN | DISCHARGE | DEAFNESS | REDNESS AND SWELLING IN OUTER EAR | SWOLLEN GLANDS | | REDNESS AND SWELLING IN EAR CANAL | SCALY SKIN IN AND AROUND EAR | ITCHINESS | FEELING OF PRESSURE | | TENDERNESS MOVING THE EAR | TENDERNESS MOVING THE JAW | DIZZINESS | OTHER:................................			
	6. Consult the General Practitioner for advice and detail the prescribed eardrops, and or analgesia and the dosage:			
	7. Ensure the application of the ear drops is as follows: • gently remove any discharge, earwax or debris from the affected outer ear using a twist of cotton wool • warm the ear drops by holding them in your hands for a few minutes, as cold ear drops can cause a feeling of dizziness • the patient should be lying on their side with the affected ear facing up • the ear drops should be applied directly into the external ear canal • gently push and pull the ear for about 30 seconds to work the drops in and allow any trapped air out • the patient should remain lying down for 3 to 5 minutes to ensure that the ear drops do not come out of the ear canal • leave the ear canal open to dry			

Copyright © 2020 Planning For Care Limited

CARE PLAN: Ear Infection Outer Ear

This care plan must be reviewed monthly (or more often if required) and each action must be signed and dated

Patient's Issues and Objectives	Consultation Assessment and Plan	Signature	Date	Review Date
	8. Ensure the ear is kept dry when the patient is showering or bathing.			
	9. Detail any issues the patient may have with the treatment and the agreed plan to address these:			
	10. Monitor the effects of the prescribed eardrops and liaise with the General Practitioner as necessary.			

Name	Patient/Relative Signature	Date

Copyright © 2020 Planning For Care Limited

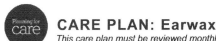

CARE PLAN: Earwax

This care plan must be reviewed monthly (or more often if required) and each action must be signed and dated

Earwax is produced by sebaceous glands in the outer third of the ear canal, the purpose of this natural wax is to protect the ear from damage and infections. Normally, a small amount of wax accumulates, then dries up and falls out of the ear canal, carrying with it unwanted dust or sand particles. It helps to coat the skin of the ear canal where it acts as a temporary water repellent, it is slightly acidic and has antibacterial properties. The colour of earwax varies depending upon its composition. Glandular secretions, sloughed skin cells, normal bacteria present on the surface of the canal, and water may all be present in earwax. The quantity made varies greatly from person to person. Some people form blockages and plugs of earwax in their ear canal, and hearing aids or earplugs can increase the chance of this, as they stop it falling out of the ear naturally. A hard plug of earwax can cause dulled hearing and sometimes 'ringing in the ear', tinnitus, or even a mild dizziness, vertigo. Eardrops alone will often clear a plug of earwax. Ear irrigation may be needed if the eardrops do not work. Irrigating the ear with water will usually clear plugs of earwax. But, it often only works if the plug of earwax has been softened.

Patient's Issues and Objectives	Consultation Assessment and Plan	Signature	Date	Review Date
Earwax To avoid a build up of wax and prevent a blockage of earwax and to reassure the patient	1. Discuss the presence of earwax with the patient and, or relative and agree the plan of care.			
	2. Note the patient's and, or relative's understanding of the issue and any concerns or anxieties they have:			
	3. Note the patient's past history of issues with earwax:			
	4. Which ear is affected:	LEFT	RIGHT	BOTH				
	5. Highlight the symptoms evident or experienced: 	HEARING LOSS	DULLED HEARING	EAR ACHE	TINNITUS	DIZZINESS	ITCHINESS	VERTIGO | OTHER			
	6. Consult with the General Practitioner for advice.			
	7. Note the General Practitioners advice and, or the prescribed eardrops and dosage:			
	8. Ensure that the eardrops are at room temperature when they are instilled into the affected ear. The patient should lie down with the affected ear facing upwards for a few minutes to allow the eardrops to soak into the wax and soften it.			
	9. Detail any issues the patient may have with the treatment and the agreed plan to address these:			
	10. Monitor the effects of the prescribed eardrops.			

Copyright © 2020 Planning For Care Limited

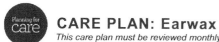

CARE PLAN: Earwax

This care plan must be reviewed monthly (or more often if required) and each action must be signed and dated

Patient's Issues and Objectives	Consultation Assessment and Plan	Signature	Date	Review Date
	11. Liaise with the General Practitioner when the course of treatment is completed, where the drops alone have not removed the wax the General Practitioner may prescribe further treatment, another course of eardrops or irrigation.			

Name	Patient/Relative Signature	Date

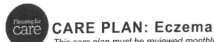

CARE PLAN: Eczema

This care plan must be reviewed monthly (or more often if required) and each action must be signed and dated

There are many types of eczema, which have different causes. The most common types are atopic dermatitis and contact dermatitis, either allergic or irritant. Atopic dermatitis often occurs in people who suffer from allergies. It can run in families and often occurs alongside other conditions such as asthma and hay fever. Allergic contact dermatitis occurs when the skin becomes sensitised to something over a period of time and an allergic reaction occurs on re-exposure. Irritant contact dermatitis occurs when the skin comes in contact with something that strips away its natural oils and makes the skin red, dry, cracked and itchy. In mild cases, eczema is nothing more than a slightly irritating patch of sore skin, but in severe cases extensive areas of skin may become inflamed and unbearably itchy.

Patient's Issues and Objectives	Consultation Assessment and Plan	Signature	Date	Review Date
Eczema Promotion and maintenance of healthy skin	1. Discuss the condition with the patient and/or relative and agree the plan of care.			
	2. Note the patient's and, or relative's understanding of the condition and any concerns or anxieties they have:			
	3. Note any past history of eczema and the treatment received:			
	4. Highlight and discuss with the patient and/or relatives any possible contributing factor or triggers: • Irritants, soap, detergents, shampoo, bubble bath • Environmental factors or allergens, cold weather, dampness, dust mites, pet fur, pollen and mould • Food allergies, cow milk, eggs, peanuts, soya, wheat • Certain materials worn next to the skin wool and synthetic fabrics • Hormonal • Skin infections			
	5. Note, where possible, the plan of care to reduce or eliminate any contributing factors:			
	6. Highlight the area(s) affected by eczema: | BACK OF KNEE | FRONT OF KNEE | OUTSIDE OF ELBOWS| AROUND THE NECK | HANDS | CHEEKS | SCALP |			

Copyright © 2020 Planning For Care Limited

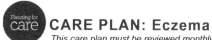

CARE PLAN: Eczema

This care plan must be reviewed monthly (or more often if required) and each action must be signed and dated

Patient's Issues and Objectives	Consultation Assessment and Plan	Signature	Date	Review Date
	7. Consult with the patient's General Practitioner.			
	8. Note the prescribed medication dosage and treatment regime:			
	9. Identify any issues the patient may have with the application of creams:			
	10. Observe for any of the following signs of infection, and seek medical assistance if suspected: • eczema getting a lot worse • fluid oozing from the skin • a yellow crust on the skin surface or small yellowish-white spots appearing in the eczema • the skin becoming swollen and sore • a high temperature, fever, and generally feeling unwell			
	....			

Name	Patient/Relative Signature	Date

Copyright © 2020 Planning For Care Limited

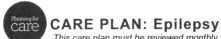

CARE PLAN: Epilepsy

This care plan must be reviewed monthly (or more often if required) and each action must be signed and dated

When nerve cells in the brain fire electrical impulses at a rate of up to four times higher than normal, this causes a sort of electrical storm in the brain, known as a seizure. A pattern of repeated seizures is referred to as epilepsy. Known causes include head injuries, brain tumors, lead poisoning, alcohol abuse, drug abuse, mal development of the brain, genetic and infectious illnesses. But in fully half of cases, no cause can be found. Medication controls seizures for the majority of patients. The severity of the seizures can differ. Some people simply experience a 'trance-like' state for a few seconds or minutes, while others lose consciousness and have convulsions, uncontrollable shaking. Status epilepticus is a seizure that lasts longer than 30 minutes or a series of seizures where the person does not regain consciousness in between. If a seizure lasts longer than five minutes medical advice must be taken.

Patient's Issues and Objectives	Consultation Assessment and Plan	Signature	Date	Review Date
Epilepsy To effectively manage epilepsy and promote health and safety	1. Discuss the condition with the patient and, or relative and agree the plan of care.			
	2. Note the patient's and, or relative's understanding of the condition and any concerns or anxieties they have:			
	3. Note details of any past history of epilepsy, the frequency of seizures, the duration and treatment:			
	4. Ask the patient if they experience a warning sign that a seizure is on its way. This is known as an aura.			
	5. Highlight any auras previously experienced which may include: | FEELING THE WORLD HAS BECOME DREAMLIKE | BODY SUDDENLY FEELS STRANGE | FEELING OF DÉJÀ VU | | SENSE OF ANXIETY | SENSE OF FEAR | STRANGE SMELL | STRANGE TASTE | SPECIFY:............................			
	6. Note the prescribed medication dosage and frequency:			
	7. Highlight the type of seizure most commonly experienced: • Grand Mal which is losing consciousness, involuntary shaking, rigidity and convulsions • Petit Mal which is a trance like state			
	8. When alerted by an aura or epileptic seizure, ensure the patient's safety is maintained. Clear an area around them. Put them in the recovery position, lying on their side with their airway clear. Never put anything in the patient's mouth during an attack, stay with them until consciousness is regained. If a seizure lasts longer than five minutes medical advice must be sought.			

Copyright © 2020 Planning For Care Limited

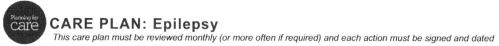

CARE PLAN: Epilepsy

This care plan must be reviewed monthly (or more often if required) and each action must be signed and dated

Patient's Issues and Objectives	Consultation Assessment and Plan	Signature	Date	Review Date
	9. Document in the patient's notes the occurrence and the length of time of the seizure.			

	10. Continue to observe until fully conscious, assessing the level of consciousness and record:
	  a. Eye response
	  b. Verbal response
	  c. Motor response			

	11. Ensure bloods are checked as requested by the General Practitioner.			
	12. Liaise with the patient's General Practitioner as required.			

Name	Patient/Relative Signature	Date

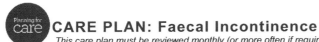

CARE PLAN: Faecal Incontinence

This care plan must be reviewed monthly (or more often if required) and each action must be signed and dated

Incontinence is the inability to control excretions. Faecal incontinence is the inability to control bowel movements, causing faeces to leak unexpectedly from the rectum. Faecal incontinence is a symptom of an underlying problem or medical condition. Many cases are caused by diarrhoea, constipation, or weakening of the muscle that controls the opening of the anus. It can also be caused by long-term conditions such as diabetes, multiple sclerosis and dementia.

Patient's Issues and Objectives	Consultation Assessment and Plan	Signature	Date	Review Date
Faecal Incontinence To promote continence where possible To effectively manage the condition	1. Discuss the condition sensitively with the patient and, or relative and agree the plan of care.			
	2. Note the patient's and, or relative's understanding of the condition and any concerns or anxieties they have:			
	3. Note the past medical history of any bowel issues, when diagnosed, the diagnosis and any treatment received:			
	4. Highlight any factors which may be contributing to the condition: | DISORIENTATION | CONFUSION | DEMENTIA | DEPRESSION | NEEDS HELP UNDRESSING | MOBILITY SLOW | | POOR MOBILITY | TOTAL IMMOBILITY | POOR DEXTERITY | OTHER:………			
	5. Specify the agreed care plan to assist with or improve any of the contributing factors:			
	6. Note the patient's normal bowel function: Frequency: Time of day:			
	7. Specify the agreed plan of care based on the outcome of the patient's continence assessment: Day: Night:			

Copyright © 2020 Planning For Care Limited

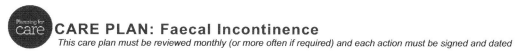

CARE PLAN: Faecal Incontinence

This care plan must be reviewed monthly (or more often if required) and each action must be signed and dated

Patient's Issues and Objectives	Consultation Assessment and Plan	Signature	Date	Review Date
	8. Note the prescribed medication, dosage and frequency:			
	9. Encourage an adequate fluid intake 1500-2000mls per day, explaining the importance of this.			
	10. Identify any issues the patient has regarding taking sufficient fluids and the agreed plan to address them:			
	11. Encourage a well-balanced, high fibre diet.			
	12. Observe the patient's skin integrity and maintain excellent personal hygiene standards.			
	13. Monitor the issue and liaise with General Practitioner as required.			

Name	Patient/Relative Signature	Date

Copyright © 2020 Planning For Care Limited

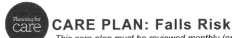

CARE PLAN: Falls Risk

This care plan must be reviewed monthly (or more often if required) and each action must be signed and dated

Falls represent the most frequent cause of injury in the elderly population. This can be due to one or more risk factors. The more risks present the greater the risk of falls. Older people are more likely to have a fall because they may have balance problems and muscle weakness, poor vision and a health condition, such as heart disease, dementia or low blood pressure, hypotension, which can lead to dizziness and a brief loss of consciousness. On admission a falls risk assessment and questionnaire must be completed. It incorporates information from the pre admission enquiry form, Care Needs Assessment Plan, the patient and their relative. This must be reviewed monthly. Many elderly patients prefer to wear slippers for comfort, however, it is of utmost importance that they wear appropriate well fitting and supportive footwear when mobilising to minimise the risk of falls.

Patient's Issues and Objectives	Consultation Assessment and Plan	Signature	Date	Review Date
High risk of falling To minimise the risk of falling and promote a safe environment	1. Discuss the issue with the patient and, or relative and agree the plan of care.			
	2. Discuss with the patient and, or relative the falls risk assessment and the factors causing an increased risk of falls. Note any concerns or anxieties they have:			
	3. Note if the patient has any memory issues or issues with understanding:			
	4. Assess if there is a pattern of when and why previous falls have occurred.			
	5. Note any medication which may increase the risk of falls:			
	6. Highlight the agreed plan of care to address the risk of falls: • ensure the environment is free from obstacles and obstructions • ensure the patient's buzzer is within reach • where the patient has impaired eyesight encourage them to wear prescribed glasses • where the patient has impaired hearing encourage them to wear their hearing aid • ensure the patient's room is well lit • encourage the patient to wear suitable, well-fitting footwear • raised toilet seat has been assessed as being a benefit to the patient • review medication			
	7. Note the agreed plan of care for mobilising or addressing any issues regarding the patient's safety:			

Copyright © 2020 Planning For Care Limited

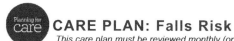

CARE PLAN: Falls Risk

This care plan must be reviewed monthly (or more often if required) and each action must be signed and dated

Patient's Issues and Objectives	Consultation Assessment and Plan	Signature	Date	Review Date
	8. Highlight if a form of restraint has been assessed as beneficial to the patient and agreed as part of the plan of care: | PRESSURE MAT | LAP STRAP | SPECIALISED CHAIR | BED RAILS |			
	9. Ensure all equipment is routinely checked to be safe and in good working order, such as walking aids, wheelchairs, commodes and arm chairs.			
	10. Review the falls risk assessment monthly and review the care plan accordingly.			
	11. Where the patient has had more than one fall, consider commencing a falls diary to identify the times of the day and the circumstances of any fall.			
	12. Liaise with the patient's General Practitioner where appropriate.			

Name	Patient/Relative Signature	Date

Copyright © 2020 Planning For Care Limited

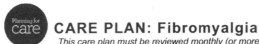

CARE PLAN: Fibromyalgia

This care plan must be reviewed monthly (or more often if required) and each action must be signed and dated

Fibromyalgia means pain coming from the muscles and fibrous tissues such as tendons and ligaments. The main symptoms are generalised pain felt in many areas of the body, and tiredness, the neck and back are often the most painful. The severity of the pain can vary from day to day and person to person, and may be made worse by stress, cold, or activity. Other symptoms can include increased sensitivity to pain, fatigue, muscle stiffness, difficulty sleeping, problems with mental processes, headaches, irritable bowel syndrome, irritable bladder, restless legs syndrome, pins and needles in fingers or toes, feeling too hot or too cold, depression or anxiety. Symptoms sometimes begin after a physical trauma, surgery, infection or significant psychological stress. In other cases, symptoms gradually accumulate with no single triggering event. The exact cause is unknown, but it is thought to be related to abnormal levels of certain chemicals in the brain, and changes in the way the central nervous system processes pain messages. While there is no cure for fibromyalgia, a variety of medications can help control symptoms. Exercise, relaxation and stress-reduction measures also may help.

Patient's Issues and Objectives	Consultation Assessment and Plan	Signature	Date	Review Date
Fibromyalgia To promote effective management of the condition To maintain an optimal level of independence and lifestyle	1. Discuss the condition with the patient and, or relative and agree the plan of care.			
	2. Note the patient's and, or relative's understanding of the condition and any concerns or anxieties they have:			
	3. Note the past medical history of Fibromyalgia, when it was diagnosed and any treatment received:			
	4. Highlight the severity of pain experienced by the patient: | MILD | INTERMITTENT | MODERATE | SEVERE | VARIES |			
	5. Note the precise location(s) of pain, if it radiates and where it radiates to:			
	6. **Highlight any other symptoms experienced by the patient:** | INCREASED SENSITIVITY TO PAIN | FATIGUE | MUSCLE STIFFNESS | DIZZINESS | ANXIETY | IRRITABLE BLADDER | | FEELING TOO HOT OR COLD | IRRITABLE BOWEL SYNDROME | RESTLESS LEGS | LACK OF CONCENTRATION | | MEMORY ISSUES | DEPRESSION | PINS AND NEEDLES | HEADACHES | SPECIFY:...			
	7. Discuss with the patient and, or relative the benefit of exercising, relaxation and stress reduction and detail the agreed plan:			
	8. Note any emotional or psychological issues the patient has due to his or her condition:			

Copyright © 2020 Planning For Care Limited

CARE PLAN: Fibromyalgia

This care plan must be reviewed monthly (or more often if required) and each action must be signed and dated

Patient's Issues and Objectives	Consultation Assessment and Plan	Signature	Date	Review Date
	9. Note any issues the patient has with the activities of daily living and the agreed plan to address them:			
	10. Note any other issues the patient has and the agreed plan to address them:			
	11. Note the prescribed medication, dose and frequency for the symptoms experienced by the patient:			
	12. Monitor the patient's condition and consult with the General Practitioner if required.			

Name	Patient/Relative Signature	Date

Copyright © 2020 Planning For Care Limited

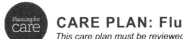

CARE PLAN: Flu

This care plan must be reviewed monthly (or more often if required) and each action must be signed and dated

Flu is an infectious viral illness spread by coughs and sneezes. It's not the same as the common cold, it is caused by a different group of viruses. Symptoms tend to be more severe and last longer. They peak after two to three days and usually last for a week or so. The infectious period is a day before the symptoms start and continues for a further five or six days. Elderly people and anyone with certain long-term medical conditions are more likely to have a bad case of flu and are also more likely to develop a serious complication such as a chest infection. Occasionally, this chest infection can become serious and develop into pneumonia.

Patient's Issues and Objectives	Consultation Assessment and Plan	Signature	Date	Review Date
Influenza To promote the healing process, to prevent recurrence, and to reassure the patient	1. Discuss the condition with the patient and, or relative and agree the plan of care.			
	2. Note the patient's and, or relative's understanding of the condition and any concerns or anxieties they have:			
	3. Highlight the symptoms experienced by the patient:	SUDDEN FEVER	DRY COUGH	CHESTY COUGH
HEADACHE	TIREDNESS	CHILLS	LIMB PAIN	JOINT PAIN	ACHING MUSCLES	DIARRHOEA	UPSET STOMACH
SORE THROAT	RUNNY NOSE	BLOCKED NOSE	SNEEZING	LOSS OF APPETITE	DIFFICULTY SLEEPING | OTHER:..			
	4. Record and monitor the patient's temperature, pulse, respirations, and blood pressure in the patient's notes, daily or more frequently as required.			
	5. Consult with the General Practitioner for advice.			
	6. Note any prescribed medication and dosage:			
	7. Explain that the flu is contagious and stress the importance of good hand washing and infection control.			
	8. Note any assistance the patient may require to ensure the infection is not passed on to others:			
	9. Highlight the individual agreed plan of care: • encourage the patient to sit up in a chair for periods throughout the day • encourage the patient to be in a upright sitting position when in bed • encourage the patient to eat and drink adequate fluids			

Copyright © 2020 Planning For Care Limited

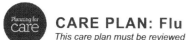

CARE PLAN: Flu

This care plan must be reviewed monthly (or more often if required) and each action must be signed and dated

Patient's Issues and Objectives	Consultation Assessment and Plan	Signature	Date	Review Date
	10. Note any additional agreed plan of care required for the safety, adequate hydration, postural drainage, comfort, and mental stimulation of the patient:			
	11. Consult the General Practitioner if the patient shows any signs of the following: • symptoms persist for more than three weeks • chest pain or difficulty breathing, signs of chest infection or pneumonia • severe swelling of the lymph nodes, glands • confusion, disorientation, drowsiness • coughing up blood or blood-stained phlegm			
	....			

Name	Patient/Relative Signature	Date

Copyright © 2020 Planning For Care Limited

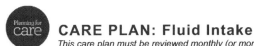

CARE PLAN: Fluid Intake

This care plan must be reviewed monthly (or more often if required) and each action must be signed and dated

Water is essential for life and it is very important to get the right amount of fluid to be healthy. To function properly, all the cells and organs of the body need water. It is also used to lubricate the joints, protect the spinal cord and other sensitive tissues, regulate body temperature, and assist the passage of food through the intestines. Although some of the water required by the body is obtained through foods with a high water content, soups, tomatoes, and oranges, the majority is gained through drinking water and other beverages. During every day functioning, water is lost by the body, and this needs to be replaced. It is noticeable that we lose water through activities such as sweating and urination, but water is even lost when breathing. Drinking water is the best source of fluid for the body. Beverages such as milk and juices are also decent sources of fluid. An adequate fluid intake is regarded as between 1500mls and 2000mls.

Patient's Issues and Objectives	Consultation Assessment and Plan	Signature	Date	Review Date
Fluid Intake To maintain adequate hydration, and to maintain optimal health	1. Discuss the patient's fluid intake requirements with the patient and, or relative and agree the plan of care.			
	2. Detail any issues the patient has with drinking fluids: • Swallowing issues • Physical disability unable to lift the fluids independently to drink • Weakness unable to lift the fluids independently to drink • Poor memory and understanding • Believing drinking less will mean reduced toilet visits • Mental health issues			
	3. Highlight the preferred or recommended consistency of fluids: | NORMAL | THICKENED FLUIDS ONE SCOOP | | THICKENED FLUIDS TWO SCOOPS |................................			
	4. Highlight how frequently the patient likes to drink. | LIKES TO HAVE A DRINK BESIDE THEM AT ALL TIMES | | LIKES TO HAVE A DRINK HOURLY | LIKES TO HAVE A DRINK EVERY TWO HOURS | RELUCTANT TO DRINK |................................			
	5. Highlight the patient preferred cup or specialised drinking aid: | CUP AND SAUCER | CUP | MUG | | TWO HANDLED BEAKER | TWO HANDLED BEAKER WITH LID | TWO HANDLED BEAKER WITH STRAW ACCESS | | NO HANDLED BEAKER WITH SPOUT |................................			
	6. Highlight what assistance the patient needs choosing drinks: | INDEPENDENT | NEEDS ENCOURAGEMENT | | NEEDS HELP | VARIES DAILY | CONSULT RELATIVE TO CHOOSE PATIENT'S PREFERENCES FROM MENU |			
	7. Note the patient's favourite drinks:			

Copyright © 2020 Planning For Care Limited

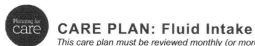

CARE PLAN: Fluid Intake

This care plan must be reviewed monthly (or more often if required) and each action must be signed and dated

Patient's Issues and Objectives	Consultation Assessment and Plan	Signature	Date	Review Date
	8. Highlight the assistance the patient requires for drinking: | INDEPENDENT | NEEDS ENCOURAGEMENT | | NEEDS ASSISTANCE | ASSESS NEEDS DAILY |			

Name	Patient/Relative Signature	Date

Copyright © 2020 Planning For Care Limited

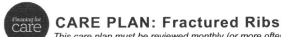

CARE PLAN: Fractured Ribs

This care plan must be reviewed monthly (or more often if required) and each action must be signed and dated

A rib fracture is a crack or break in one of the bones of the rib cage. The most common cause is a direct blow to the chest, often from a car accident or a fall. Coughing hard can also cause a rib to fracture, this is more likely to happen if bones are weak, such as with osteoporosis or cancer. Fractured, broken or bruised ribs will feel painful with every intake of breath or cough, this can result in shallow breathing to avoid pain, which can result in a chest Infection or pneumonia. Swelling and tenderness around the injured area can be experienced, as well as bruising to the skin. A doctor may diagnose the fracture through physical examination or X-ray, however a fractured rib sometimes does not show up. Most rib injuries heal well within 6 weeks, with no problems. Complications such as a pneumothorax, air in the lung cavity, haemothorax, blood in the lung cavity, atelectasis, collapse of the lung, pneumonia, chest infection or lung contusions can occur.

Patient's Issues and Objectives	Consultation Assessment and Plan	Signature	Date	Review Date
Fractured Ribs To minimise pain and discomfort to promote effective management of the condition To maintain an optimal level of independence and lifestyle	1. Discuss the condition with the patient and, or relative and agree the plan of care.			
	2. Note the patient's and, or relative's understanding of the condition and any concerns or anxieties they have:			
	3. Note the extent and area of the fracture(s):			
	4. Pain is the main symptom, note the level of pain and the prescribed analgesia, the frequency and dose:			
	5. Note in detail any assistance, the patient requires with the activities of daily living and the agreed plan to address them:			
	6. Encourage the patient to breathe properly, using the full expanse of their lungs.			

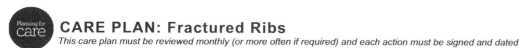

CARE PLAN: Fractured Ribs

This care plan must be reviewed monthly (or more often if required) and each action must be signed and dated

Patient's Issues and Objectives	Consultation Assessment and Plan	Signature	Date	Review Date
	7. Consult the GP if the patient shows signs of the following, as this can indicate complications: • increasing shortness of breath • increasing chest pain • pain in the abdomen or shoulder • coughing up blood, and, or yellow or green mucous • high temperature, fever of 38C (100.4F) or above			

Name	Patient/Relative Signature	Date

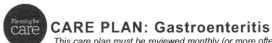

CARE PLAN: Gastroenteritis

This care plan must be reviewed monthly (or more often if required) and each action must be signed and dated

Gastroenteritis is an infection of the stomach and bowel. The most common symptoms are repeated episodes of diarrhoea, three or more episodes within the space of twenty four hours, and vomiting. Gastroenteritis can be caused by a virus such as the norovirus, or by a number of different types of bacteria. Typically, bacterial gastroenteritis develops as a result of food poisoning. These infections can interfere with the absorption of water and salts from the contents of the intestines into the body, which is why the most common symptom of gastroenteritis is watery diarrhoea and why there is a high risk of dehydration.

Patient's Issues and Objectives	Consultation Assessment and Plan	Signature	Date	Review Date
Gastroenteritis To effectively promote recovery and alleviate any concerns To prevent cross infection or contamination	1. Discuss the infection with the patient and, or relative and agree the plan of care.			
	2. Explain the importance of infection control and barrier nursing measures, which will be implemented.			
	3. Note the patient's and, or relative's understanding of the condition and any concerns they have:			
	4. Highlight the symptoms the patient has: | DIARRHOEA | FEELING SICK | LOSS OF APPETITE | HEADACHES | | STOMACH CRAMPS | ACHING LIMBS | HIGH TEMPERATURE |................			
	5. Note the agreed plan of care for any issues the patient has, and any infection control issues:			
	6. Encourage the patient to stay in his, or her bedroom whilst symptomatic and for 48 hours after the last symptom.			
	7. Highlight the patient's preferences for recreation or mental stimulation and detail choices: | TELEVISION | DVDS | RADIO MUSIC | RADIO TALK SHOWS | READING | CROSSWORDS|................			
	8. Ensure good hand-washing techniques are used by all staff, patient and visitors.			
	9. Gloves and apron must be worn by all staff when giving personal care to the patient, removed before leaving the patient's room and put into a clinical waste bag.			
	10. All clothing must be put into alginate bags and sealed before leaving the bedroom.			
	11. Encourage the patient to use the en suite toilet, where possible or a designated commode.			
	12. Environmental cleaning must be increased paying particular attention to toilet areas, bathrooms, door handles and support hand rails, for the duration of the outbreak.			
	13. Obtain a stool specimen and note the date it was sent to the laboratory:			

Copyright © 2020 Planning For Care Limited

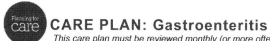

CARE PLAN: Gastroenteritis

This care plan must be reviewed monthly (or more often if required) and each action must be signed and dated

Patient's Issues and Objectives	Consultation Assessment and Plan	Signature	Date	Review Date
	14. Record in the notes the result of the stool specimen.			
	15. The person in charge must inform Public Health, Infection Control Department if 2 patients or more have the infection.			
	16. Encourage sufficient clear fluid intake 2000mls per day for first 24 hours and thereafter 2000mls per day of any fluids, introducing light diet as tolerated.			
	17. Note if insufficient fluids are being taken and commence a fluid balance chart:			
	18. Monitor the patient's skin integrity.			
	19. Note prescribed barrier cream and apply as per protocol:			
	20. Monitor the patient's condition and liaise with General Practitioner and or infection control as required.			
	....			

Name	Patient/Relative Signature	Date

Copyright © 2020 Planning For Care Limited

CARE PLAN: Generalised Anxiety Disorder

This care plan must be reviewed monthly (or more often if required) and each action must be signed and dated

Anxiety disorders include generalised anxiety disorder, social anxiety disorder, post-traumatic stress disorder, panic disorder, obsessive-compulsive disorder and body dysmorphic disorder. Although anxiety disorders vary in their severity, they are associated with long-term disability and can have a lifelong course of relapse and remission. Generalised Anxiety Disorder, GAD, can cause both psychological and physical symptoms. These symptoms vary from person to person, but can include feeling restless, irritable or worried, difficulty concentrating or sleeping, and feeling "on edge". The physical symptoms can include pins and needles, headache, dizziness, tiredness, palpitations, muscle aches and tension, dry mouth, excessive sweating, shortness of breath, stomach ache, feeling sick, or shaking. Several factors can cause anxiety, these may include over activity in areas of the brain, an imbalance of chemicals serotonin and noradrenaline, a family history of anxiety, a past history of stressful or traumatic experiences, having a painful long-term health condition, such as arthritis, or a history of drug or alcohol misuse.

Patient's Issues and Objectives	Consultation Assessment and Plan	Signature	Date	Review Date
Generalised Anxiety Disorder To develop an awareness of any specific causes To calm, comfort and alleviate anxiety, and minimise distress	1. Discuss the issues with the patient and, or relative and agree the plan of care.			
	2. Note the past medical history of the anxiety disorder, when it was diagnosed, and any treatment received:			
	3. Describe the circumstances physical or psychological which may lead to the patient feeling anxious:			
	4. Describe in detail the way in which the patient presents himself, or herself as being anxious:			
	5. Highlight the symptoms the patient experiences: | RESTLESS | IRRITABLE | WORRIED | DIFFICULTY CONCENRATING | DIFFICULTY SLEEPING | MUSCLE ACHES | TENSION | | FEELING ON EDGE | DIZZINESS | TIREDNESS | PALPITATIONS | HEADACHE | TREMBLING | STOMACH ACHE | HEADACHE | | FEELING SICK | DRY MOUTH | EXCESSIVE SWEATING | SHORTNESS OF BREATH | PINS AND NEEDLES | SHAKING | OTHER:			
	6. Specify where possible the agreed plan to comfort, reassure or calm the patient, note any phrases which may help:			

Copyright © 2020 Planning For Care Limited

CARE PLAN: Generalised Anxiety Disorder
This care plan must be reviewed monthly (or more often if required) and each action must be signed and dated

Patient's Issues and Objectives	Consultation Assessment and Plan	Signature	Date	Review Date
	7. Note any issues the patient has with the activities of daily living, due to the anxiety, and the agreed plan to address them:			
	8. Note the prescribed medication, dose and frequency for the symptoms experienced by the patient:			
	9. If necessary, give and record the prescribed PRN (Pro Re Nata) medication as required, following the Care Home's protocol. Monitor the effects and any side effects of the medication.			
	10. Liaise with the patient's General Practitioner and or Psychogeriatrician as appropriate.			

Name	Patient/Relative Signature	Date

Copyright © 2020 Planning For Care Limited

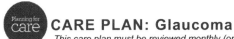

CARE PLAN: Glaucoma

This care plan must be reviewed monthly (or more often if required) and each action must be signed and dated

Glaucoma occurs when the drainage tubes, trabecular meshwork, within the eye become blocked. This prevents eye fluid, aqueous humour, from draining properly. When the fluid cannot drain properly, pressure builds up. This is called intraocular pressure. This results in damage to the optic nerve, which can lead to blindness. Glaucoma often affects both eyes in varying degrees. If it is diagnosed early enough, further damage to vision can be prevented.

Patient's Issues and Objectives	Consultation Assessment and Plan	Signature	Date	Review Date
Glaucoma Increase in intraocular pressure To effectively manage the condition and maintain optimal vision	1. Discuss the condition with the patient and, or relative and agree the plan of care.			
	2. Reassure the patient and, or relative that glaucoma is a disease that can generally be controlled. Treatment may involve the use of eye drops or surgery which can prevent any further nerve damage and visual loss.			
	3. Note any concerns the patient and/or the relative has:			
	4. Highlight the degree of visual impairment: | REGISTERED BLIND | PARTIALLY SIGHTED | POOR WITH GLASSES | | GOOD WITH GLASSES |............			
	5. Note the previous history of the disease and treatment:			
	6. Note the prescribed eye drops, dose and frequency:			
	7. Detail any issues the patient has with any of the activities of daily living as a result of the visual impairment, and the agreed plan to address them:............			
	8. Highlight any aids which may assist the patient, or improve his or her quality of life: | PLATE GUARDS | SPECIALISED CUTLERY | NON SLIP MAT FOR PLATE | MAGNIFYING GLASS | MUSIC SYSTEM | | RADIO | TALKING BOOK | TALKING NEWSPAPER | OTHER:............			

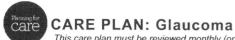

CARE PLAN: Glaucoma

This care plan must be reviewed monthly (or more often if required) and each action must be signed and dated

Patient's Issues and Objectives	Consultation Assessment and Plan	Signature	Date	Review Date
	9. Detail any issues the patient has with safety as a result of the visual impairment, and the agreed plan to address this:..			
	10. Encourage the patient to wear prescribed glasses.			
	11. Specify any issues the patient has with wearing glasses:			
	12. Monitor the condition and report any change in eyesight or discomfort of eyes and refer to ophthalmologist immediately.			
	13. Ensure the patient has regular annual eye examinations.			
	....			

Name	Patient/Relative Signature	Date

Copyright © 2020 Planning For Care Limited

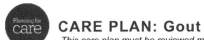

CARE PLAN: Gout
This care plan must be reviewed monthly (or more often if required) and each action must be signed and dated

Gout is a disease that results from an overload of uric acid in the body, this leads to the formation of tiny crystals of urate that deposit in tissues of the body. When crystals form in the joints, it causes recurring attacks of joint inflammation, arthritis. Gout is a painful chronic and progressive disease. Chronic gout can lead to deposits of hard lumps of uric acid in the tissues, particularly in and around the joints that may cause joint destruction, decreased kidney function, and kidney stones.

Patient's Issues and Objectives	Consultation Assessment and Plan	Signature	Date	Review Date
Gout	1. Discuss the condition with the patient and, or relative and agree the plan of care.			
	2. Note the patient's and, or relative's understanding of the condition and any concerns or anxieties they have:			
To minimise the pain and discomfort and prevent the recurrence of gout	3. Note any previous episodes of gout and what measures have been taken to improve the condition:			
	4. Highlight the contributing factors which may be causing the gout: • Obesity • High blood pressure • Diabetes • having a close relative with gout • kidney problems • eating foods that cause a build-up of uric acid, such as red meat, offal and seafood • excessive alcohol			
	5. Highlight the symptoms experienced by the patient: • severe pain in one or more joints • the joint feeling hot and very tender • swelling in and around the affected joint • red, shiny skin over the affected joint			
	6. Note the area(s) affected by gout:			
	7. Consult the General Practitioner for advice.			

Copyright © 2020 Planning For Care Limited

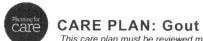

CARE PLAN: Gout

This care plan must be reviewed monthly (or more often if required) and each action must be signed and dated

Patient's Issues and Objectives	Consultation Assessment and Plan	Signature	Date	Review Date
	8. Note prescribed medication, dose and frequency:			
	9. Advise the patient to avoid beef, pork, lamb, seafood, beer and bread. Explain the benefits of foods with a low purine content.			
	10. Encourage adequate fluid intake 1500mls - 2000mls per day and monitor the intake.			
	11. Note if the patient has issues drinking an adequate fluid intake and specify any assistance required:			
	12. Encourage the patient to avoid alcohol.			
	13. Monitor the condition for improvement and for pain control and liaise with the General Practitioner as required.			
	....			

Name	Patient/Relative Signature	Date

Copyright © 2020 Planning For Care Limited

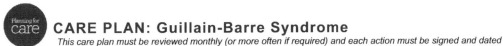

CARE PLAN: Guillain-Barre Syndrome
This care plan must be reviewed monthly (or more often if required) and each action must be signed and dated

Guillain-Barré syndrome is a rare condition of the peripheral nervous system. It occurs when the body's immune system attacks part of the nervous system. The exact cause is unknown, however, most people develop the condition shortly after having a viral or bacterial infection. Initially there may be pain, tingling and numbness and progressive muscle weakness, also co-ordination problems and unsteadiness. The weakness usually affects both sides of the body, and may get worse over several days. Life-threatening complications can develop during the first few weeks of the condition, such as respiratory failure, respiratory infections, heart rhythm disorders, including cardiac arrest and bowel obstruction. About 80% of people with Guillain-Barré syndrome make a full recovery, it may take several weeks in hospital and it may take a year or more to fully recover. Some people never recover and complications can include, persistent fatigue, needing assistance with walking, or unable to walk, loss of sensation, lack of co-ordination, loss of balance, muscle weakness in the arms or legs and issues with the sense of touch, often felt as a burning or tingling sensation.

Patient's Issues and Objectives	Consultation Assessment and Plan	Signature	Date	Review Date
Guillain-Barré Syndrome To promote effective management of the condition To maintain an optimal level of independence and lifestyle	1. Discuss the condition with the patient and, or relative and agree the plan of care.			
	2. Note the patient's and, or relative's understanding of the condition and any concerns or anxieties they have:			
	3. Note the past medical history of Guillain-Barré, when it was diagnosed and any treatment received:			
	4. **Highlight any symptoms experienced by the patient:** | PERSISTENT FATIGUE | PAIN | POOR MOBILITY | UNABLE TO MOBILISE | BURNING TINGLING SENSATION | | LOSS OF SENSATION | MUSCLE WEAKNESS IN ARMS | MUSCLE WEAKNESS IN LEGS | BREATHING ISSUES | | FLUCTUATIONS OF HEART RATE AND BLOOD PRESSURE | COORDINATION ISSUES | DIGESTION ISSUES | | BLADDER CONTROL ISSUES | BLURRED VISION | DOUBLE VISION |			
	5. Specify the affected areas of muscle weakness:			
	6. Note any issues the patient has with the activities of daily living and how they will be addressed:			

CARE PLAN: Guillain-Barre Syndrome

This care plan must be reviewed monthly (or more often if required) and each action must be signed and dated

Patient's Issues and Objectives	Consultation Assessment and Plan	Signature	Date	Review Date
	7. Note any issues with the patient's mobility and the agreed plan of care to address them:			
	8. Note any emotional or psychological issues the patient has due to his her condition:			
	9. Note the prescribed medication, dose and frequency:			
	10. Observe for any of the following complications and seek immediate medical assistance if suspected: • Respiratory failure • Infections • Heart rhythm disorders, including cardiac arrest • Bowel obstruction			

Name	Patient/Relative Signature	Date

CARE PLAN: Haemorrhoids
This care plan must be reviewed monthly (or more often if required) and each action must be signed and dated

Haemorrhoids, also called piles, are swollen and inflamed veins in the anus and lower rectum. Haemorrhoids may result from straining during bowel movements or from the increased pressure on these veins during pregnancy, among other causes. Haemorrhoids may be located inside the rectum, internal haemorrhoids, or they may develop under the skin around the anus, external haemorrhoids. It is important to remember that rectal bleeding or blood in the stool is never normal and while it may come from a relatively benign cause like haemorrhoids, more serious causes can be life threatening. These include bleeding from ulcers, diverticulitis, inflammatory bowel disease, and tumours. If rectal bleeding occurs, it is important to contact your health care professional or seek emergency medical care.

Patient's Issues And Objectives	Consultation Assessment and Plan	Signature	Date	Review Date
Haemorrhoids **To minimise any discomfort and reduce inflammation of haemorrhoids**	1. Discuss the condition with the patient and, or relative and agree the plan of care.			
	2. Note the patient's and, or relative's understanding of the condition and any concerns or anxieties they have:			
	3. Note the past history of haemorrhoids and the treatment prescribed:			
	4. Highlight and discuss with the patient and, or the relatives any possible contributing factors: | AGE | STRAINING DURING BOWEL MOVEMENTS | SITTING ON THE TOILET FOR LONG PERIODS | CONSTIPATION | | CHRONIC DIARRHOEA | LOW FIBRE DIET | OBESITY | PREGNANCY | PERSISTENT COUGH |....................			
	5. Highlight any symptoms experienced by the patient: | RECTAL BLEEDING | LUMP NEAR THE ANUS | ITCH OR IRRITATION AROUND ANUS | PAIN OR DISCOMFORT | | MUCOUS | SWELLING AROUND THE ANUS | OTHER:................			
	6. Highlight the agreed plan of care which may improve the contributing factors and prevent constipation: • encourage adequate fibre intake 15-25g per day • encourage adequate fluid intake 1500-2000ml per day • encourage daily exercise • administer any prescribed medication as directed by the General Practitioner			
	7. Note the patient's normal bowel function and pattern: Frequency..Time of Day...........................			

Copyright © 2020 Planning For Care Limited

CARE PLAN: Haemorrhoids

This care plan must be reviewed monthly (or more often if required) and each action must be signed and dated

Patient's Issues And Objectives	Consultation Assessment and Plan	Signature	Date	Review Date
	8. Note the prescribed medication, dosage, and treatment regime:			
	9. Note if the patient has any issues with the treatment and the agreed plan of care to address them:			
	11. Liaise with the patient's General Practitioner as required.			
	....			

Name	Patient/Relative Signature	Date

Copyright © 2020 Planning For Care Limited

CARE PLAN: Heart Attack or Myocardial Infarction (MI)

This care plan must be reviewed monthly (or more often if required) and each action must be signed and dated

Like any muscle, the heart tissues need a good supply of blood from the blood vessels, which are called the coronary arteries. When this is interrupted or does not work properly, serious illness and even death can result. A heart attack or Myocardial Infarction is when the supply of blood to the heart is suddenly blocked, usually by a blood clot. This can cause serious damage to the heart muscle. Symptoms include chest pain, usually a central crushing pain that may travel into the left arm or to the neck or jaw, and persists for more than a few minutes. Unlike angina, the pain does not subside when resting. Sometimes it can be mild and be mistaken for indigestion. Some people have a heart attack without experiencing pain, Normal symptoms also include stomach or abdominal pain, shortness of breath or difficulty breathing, nausea or vomiting, sweating, unexplained anxiety, weakness or fatigue, cold sweat or paleness, feeling light-headed or dizzy, palpitations or an abnormal heart rate.

Patient's Issues and Objectives	Consultation Assessment and Plan	Signature	Date	Review Date
Heart Attack or Myocardial Infarction To promote the effective management of the condition To maintain an optimal level of independence and lifestyle	1. Discuss the condition with the patient and, or relative and agree the plan of care.			
	2. Note the patient's and, or relative's understanding of the condition and any concerns or anxieties they have:			
	3. Note any past history of cardiac or heart issues, any symptoms experienced and treatment received:			
	4. Note the patient's blood pressure, temperature, pulse and respirations:			
	5. Highlight the symptoms the patient experienced prior to or during the heart attack: | CRUSHING CENTRAL CHEST PAIN | PAIN IN CHEST AND LEFT ARM, NECK AND JAW | VOMITING | SWEATING | | PAIN PERSISTS FOR MORE THAN A FEW MINUTES | PAIN DOES NOT SUBSIDE WITH REST | ANXIETY | NAUSEA | | PALPITATIONS | SHORTNESS OF BREATH | ABDOMINAL PAIN | FEELING LIGHTHEADED | FATIGUE | WEAKNESS | | ABNORMAL HEART RATE |			
	6. Note all investigations carried out and the severity of the heart attack, where known:			
	7. Highlight any contributing factors: | HIGH BLOOD PRESSURE | HIGH CHOLESTEROL LEVELS | OBESITY | SMOKING | DIABETES | KIDNEY DISEASE | | EXCESSIVE ALCOHOL | EXCESSIVE SALT | LACK OF EXERCISE | FAMILY HISTORY OF HEART DISEASE |			
	8. Note any agreed plan for lifestyle changes where appropriate:			

Copyright © 2020 Planning For Care Limited

CARE PLAN: Heart Attack or Myocardial Infarction (MI)

This care plan must be reviewed monthly (or more often if required) and each action must be signed and dated

Patient's Issues and Objectives	Consultation Assessment and Plan	Signature	Date	Review Date
	9. Note any issues the patient has with the activities of daily living and the agreed plan of care to address them:			
	10. Note the prescribed medication, dose and frequency and treatment regime:			
	11. Liaise with the General Practitioner as required.			

Name	Patient/Relative Signature	Date

CARE PLAN: Heart or Cardiac Failure

This care plan must be reviewed monthly (or more often if required) and each action must be signed and dated

Heart failure is when the heart loses its ability to pump enough blood efficiently around the body. It usually occurs because the heart muscle has become too weak or stiff to work properly. Breathlessness, feeling very tired and swollen legs, ankles and feet are the main symptoms of heart failure. Acute heart failure develops quickly. However, chronic heart failure is more common and develops gradually, over time. If the left ventricle of the heart fails fluid will build up in the lungs due to congestion of the vein in the lungs. If the right ventricle of the heart fails, general body vein pressure will increase and fluid will accumulate in the body, especially in the legs and in the abdominal organs, with the liver most likely to be affected. Often left ventricular failure, over time, leads to right ventricular failure, causing failure on both sides of the heart. Effective treatment for heart failure helps make the heart stronger, improves the symptoms, reduces the risk of a flare-up, and helps to enable people with the disease to live longer and fuller lives.

Patient's Issues and Objectives	Consultation Assessment and Plan	Signature	Date	Review Date
Heart or Cardiac Failure To promote the effective management of the condition To maintain an optimal level of independence and lifestyle	1. Discuss the condition with the patient and, or relative and agree the plan of care.			
	2. Note the patient's and, or relative's understanding of the condition and any concerns or anxieties they have:			
	3. Highlight the cause where known: | CORONARY HEART DISEASE | HEART VALVE DISEASE | HIGH BLOOD PRESSURE | ATRIAL FIBRILLATION | | SEVERE ANAEMIA | RAPID PULSE | PREVIOUS HEART ATTACK |............................			
	4. Note the patient's past history of cardiac failure, any symptoms experienced and any treatment received:			
	5. Highlight any contributing factors: | HIGH BLOOD PRESSURE | HIGH CHOLESTEROL LEVELS | EXCESSIVE SALT | | SMOKING | EXCESSIVE ALCOHOL | LACK OF EXERCISE | OBESITY |			
	6. Note any agreed plan for lifestyle changes, where appropriate:			
	7. Highlight the symptoms the patient is experiencing, or are evident: | BREATHLESSNESS AT REST | BREATHLESSNESS ON EXERTION | SWELLING IN ANKLES | SWELLING IN LEGS | | EXCESSIVE TIREDNESS |............................			
	8. Note the agreed plan for managing or relieving the patient's symptoms such oedema, breathlessness and fatigue:			

Copyright © 2020 Planning For Care Limited

CARE PLAN: Heart or Cardiac Failure

This care plan must be reviewed monthly (or more often if required) and each action must be signed and dated

Patient's Issues and Objectives	Consultation Assessment and Plan	Signature	Date	Review Date
	9. Note any issues the patient has with any activities of daily living and the agreed plan of care to address them:			
	10. Note the prescribed medication, dose and frequency:			
	11. Liaise with the General Practitioner as required.			

Name	Patient/Relative Signature	Date

Copyright © 2020 Planning For Care Limited

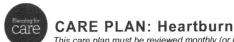

CARE PLAN: Heartburn

This care plan must be reviewed monthly (or more often if required) and each action must be signed and dated

Heartburn or Gastro-oesophageal reflux disease, GORD, occurs when the acid contents of the stomach pass backwards up into the oesophagus. Most people have stomach acid reflux at some point in their lives, either as heartburn or acid regurgitation. Frequent or severe heartburn may limit daily activities and lead to further complications such as ulcers in the oesophagus. Symptoms can include an uncomfortable feeling of burning or warmth in the chest, nausea, an acid taste in the mouth, bloating, belching, and a burning pain when drinking hot drinks. More uncommon symptoms can be a persistent cough, particularly at night, due to the refluxed acid irritating the trachea, or windpipe. Asthma symptoms of cough and wheeze can sometimes be due to acid reflux. Other mouth and throat symptoms sometimes occur such as gum problems, bad breath, sore throat, hoarseness, and a feeling of a lump in the throat. Severe chest pain can develop in some cases. With appropriate treatment, relief can be obtained from this condition.

Patient's Issues and Objectives	Consultation Assessment and Plan	Signature	Date	Review Date
Heartburn To promote effective management of the condition To maintain an optimal level of comfort and lifestyle	1. Discuss the condition with the patient and, or relative and agree the plan of care.			
	2. Note the patient's and, or relative's understanding of the condition and any concerns or anxieties they have:			
	3. Note the details of any past history of heartburn and the treatment received:			
	4. Highlight any contributing factors: | OBESITY | HIGH FAT DIET | SMOKING | EXCESSIVE ALCOHOL | EXCESSIVE COFFEE | HIATUS HERNIA | PREGNANCY |			
	5. Note any agreed plan for lifestyle changes where appropriate:			
	6. Highlight the symptoms experienced by the patient: | HEARTBURN | CHEST PAIN | ACID REFLUX | NAUSEA | BLOATING | BELCHING | PAIN WHEN SWALLOWING | COUGH | | DIFFICULTY SWALLOWING | WHEEZE | TOOTH DECAY | GUM ISSUES | BAD BREATH | HOARSENESS | LARYNGITIS |			
	7. Note the prescribed medication, dosage and frequency:			

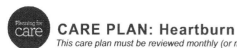

CARE PLAN: Heartburn

This care plan must be reviewed monthly (or more often if required) and each action must be signed and dated

Patient's Issues and Objectives	Consultation Assessment and Plan	Signature	Date	Review Date
	8. Highlight the agreed plan of care to avoid heartburn: • To eat smaller and more frequent meals, rather than three large meals a day • To avoid eating within three or four hours before going to bed • To avoid drinking alcohol within three or four hours before going to bed • To avoid drinking excessive amounts of alcohol • To avoid wearing tight clothes around the stomach area • To raise the head of the bed by 20cms, placing wood blocks underneath the head of the bed to raise it • To relax and reduce stress			
	9. Liaise with the patient's General Practitioner as required.			
	....			

Name	Patient/Relative Signature	Date

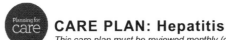

CARE PLAN: Hepatitis

This care plan must be reviewed monthly (or more often if required) and each action must be signed and dated

Hepatitis is the term used to describe inflammation of the liver. It's usually the result of a viral infection or liver damage caused by drinking alcohol. There are several different types of hepatitis. Hepatitis A, caused by the hepatitis A virus is usually caught by consuming food and drink contaminated with the faeces of an infected person. Hepatitis B is caused by the hepatitis B virus, which is spread in the blood of an infected person. Hepatitis C, is caused by the hepatitis C virus is usually spread through blood-to-blood contact with an infected person. Hepatitis D only affects people who are already infected with hepatitis B, as it needs the hepatitis B virus to be able to survive in the body. Hepatitis E is usually caused by consuming food and drink contaminated with the faeces of an infected person. Alcoholic hepatitis is caused by drinking excessive amounts of alcohol over many years. Autoimmune hepatitis is caused when the immune system attacks and damages the liver. Some types of hepatitis will pass without any serious problems, while others can be long-lasting or chronic and cause scarring or cirrhosis of the liver, loss of liver function and, in some cases, liver cancer.

Patient's Issues and Objectives	Consultation Assessment and Plan	Signature	Date	Review Date
Hepatitis To promote the effective management of the condition To maintain an optimal level of independence and lifestyle	1. Discuss the condition with the patient and, or relative and agree the plan of care.			
	2. Note the patient's and, or the relative's understanding of the condition and any concerns or anxieties they have:			
	3. Note the patient's past history of hepatitis, the cause, any symptoms experienced, and any treatment received:			
	4. Highlight the type of hepatitis the patient has: | HEPATITIS A | HEPATITIS B | HEPATITIS C | HEPATITIS D | | HEPATITIS E | ALCOHOLIC HEPATITIS | AUTOIMMUNE HEPATITIS |............			
	5. Highlight any symptoms experienced by the patient: | NO SYMPTOMS | MUSCLE PAIN | JOINT PAIN | VOMITING | | NAUSEA | HIGH TEMPERATURE | TIREDNESS | WEAKNESS | FEELING GENERALLY UNWELL | LOSS OF APPETITE | | ABDOMINAL PAIN | DARK COLOURED URINE | PALE GRAY COLOURED STOOLS | JAUNDICE YELLOWING SKIN | | YELLOWING OF THE WHITE OF THE EYES | ITCHY SKIN |............			
	6. Note the agreed plan of care to address any issues the patient has with any of the activities of daily living:			

CARE PLAN: Hepatitis

This care plan must be reviewed monthly (or more often if required) and each action must be signed and dated

Patient's Issues and Objectives	Consultation Assessment and Plan	Signature	Date	Review Date
	7. Consult the General practitioner for advice and detail any advice:			

Name	Patient/Relative Signature	Date

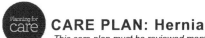

CARE PLAN: Hernia
This care plan must be reviewed monthly (or more often if required) and each action must be signed and dated

A hernia occurs when an internal part of the body pushes through a weakness in the muscle or surrounding tissue wall. In many cases, hernias cause no or very few symptoms. The lump can often be pushed back in or will disappear when lying down. Coughing or straining may make the lump appear. Hernias can occur in many different parts of the body. Inguinal and femoral hernias occur in the groin area at the top of the inner thigh, epigastric hernias occur in the abdomen, between the navel and the breastbone, umbilical hernias occur in the abdomen near the belly button, hiatus hernias occur when part of the stomach pushes upwards through an opening in the diaphragm, and incisional hernias occur when tissue protrudes through a surgical wound which has not properly healed. If the patient complains of, or experiences symptoms such as sudden, severe pain, vomiting, constipation or wind, or the hernia becomes firm or tender, or cannot be pushed back the General Practitioner should be informed immediately as it may indicate a medical emergency. These symptoms could mean that the blood supply to a section of organ or tissue trapped in the hernia has become cut off, or strangulated, or that a piece of bowel has entered the hernia and become blocked. A strangulated hernia and obstructed bowel are medical emergencies.

Patient's Issues and Objectives	Consultation Assessment and Plan	Signature	Date	Review Date
Hernia To promote effective management of the hernia To observe for any complications	1. Discuss the hernia with the patient and, or relative and agree the plan of care.			
	2. Note the patient's and, or relative's understanding of the hernia and any concerns or anxieties they have:			
	3. Note details of the past history of the hernia, when it appeared, and the type of hernia:			
	4. Note where the hernia is on the patient's body and any issues they have experienced in relation to the hernia:			
	5. Monitor the hernia daily for any signs of change.			
	6. Note the prescribed medication dosage and frequency:			
	7. Liaise with the patient's General Practitioner as required.			

Copyright © 2020 Planning For Care Limited

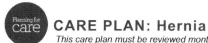

CARE PLAN: Hernia

This care plan must be reviewed monthly (or more often if required) and each action must be signed and dated

Patient's Issues and Objectives	Consultation Assessment and Plan	Signature	Date	Review Date
	8. Observe for any of the following signs or symptoms of complications, if present seek immediate medical assistance:<ul><li>sudden, severe pain</li><li>vomiting</li><li>difficulty passing stools, constipation, or wind</li><li>the hernia becomes firm or tender, or cannot be pushed back</li></ul>			

Name	Patient/Relative Signature	Date

CARE PLAN: Hiatus Hernia

This care plan must be reviewed monthly (or more often if required) and each action must be signed and dated

A hiatus hernia occurs when part of the stomach protrudes through an opening in the diaphragm muscle into the lower chest. The hernia itself may not always cause symptoms, It can cause highly irritating stomach contents, such as acid, to pass up into the oesophagus. It can cause heartburn, which is a burning feeling which rises from the upper abdomen or lower chest up towards the neck. Other common symptoms include pain in the upper abdomen and chest, nausea, an acid taste in the mouth, bloating, belching, and a burning pain when drinking hot drinks. More uncommon symptoms can be a persistent cough, particularly at night, due to the refluxed acid irritating the trachea, windpipe. Asthma symptoms of cough and wheeze can sometimes be due to acid reflux. Other mouth and throat symptoms sometimes occur such as gum problems, bad breath, sore throat, hoarseness, and a feeling of a lump in the throat. Severe chest pain can develop in some cases, and may be mistaken for a heart attack.

Patient's Issues and Objectives	Consultation Assessment and Plan	Signature	Date	Review Date
Hiatus Hernia	1. Discuss the condition with the patient and, or relative and agree the plan of care.			
	2. Note the patient's and, or relative's understanding of the condition and any concerns or anxieties they have:			
To promote effective management of the condition	3. Note details of the past history of the hiatus hernia and the treatment received:			
	4. Highlight any symptoms experienced by the patient: | HEARTBURN | CHEST PAIN | ACID REFLUX | NAUSEA | PAIN WHEN SWALLOWING | DIFFICULTY SWALLOWING | | BLOATING | BELCHING | COUGH | WHEEZE | GUM PROBLEMS | BAD BREATH | SORE THROAT | HOARSENESS |			
To maintain an optimal level of independence and lifestyle	5. Highlight the foods which aggravate the symptoms the patient experiences, and should be avoided: | CHOCOLATE | TOMATOES | FATTY FOODS | SPICY FOODS | ACIDIC FOODS | ACIDIC FRUIT JUICES |			
	6. Note the agreed plan of care to alleviate or relieve the symptoms of hiatus hernia: • to eat smaller, more frequent meals, rather than three large meals a day • to avoid lying down or going to bed for at least three hours after eating or drinking • to avoid drinking during the night • to avoid bending over or stooping, particularly after eating or drinking • to raise the head of the bed by 20cms by placing a piece of wood under it • to avoid drinking alcohol • to avoid drinking tea and coffee			

Copyright © 2020 Planning For Care Limited

140

CARE PLAN: Hiatus Hernia

This care plan must be reviewed monthly (or more often if required) and each action must be signed and dated

Patient's Issues and Objectives	Consultation Assessment and Plan	Signature	Date	Review Date
	7. Note the prescribed medication dosage and frequency:			
	8. Liaise with the patient's General Practitioner as required.			

Name	Patient/Relative Signature	Date

CARE PLAN: Huntington's Disease

This care plan must be reviewed monthly (or more often if required) and each action must be signed and dated

Huntington's disease is a degenerative disorder of certain nerve cells in the brain. The brain damage gets progressively worse over time and can affect movement, perception, awareness, thinking, judgement and behaviour. Early features can include personality changes, mood swings, fidgety movements, irritability and altered behaviour, although these are often overlooked and attributed to something else. It is a genetic disease, with no cure and its progress cannot be reversed or slowed down. The clinical features of Huntington's disease can include psychiatric problems, feeding issues, communication and abnormal movements.

Patient's Issues and Objectives	Consultation Assessment and Plan	Signature	Date	Review Date
Huntington's Disease To maintain an optimal level of independence and lifestyle	1. Discuss the condition with the patient and, or relatives and agree the plan of care.			
	2. Note the patient's and, or relative's understanding of the condition and any concerns or anxieties they have:			
	3. Note the patient's past history of the condition if available:			
	4. Highlight any issues or symptoms experienced by the patient as a result of the condition: | INVOLUNTARY JERKING | INVOLUNTARY WRITHING MOVEMENTS | MUSCLE RIGIDITY | ABNORMAL EYE MOVEMENTS | | IMPAIRED GAIT | POOR BALANCE | DIFFICULTY WITH SPEECH | DIFFICULTY SWALLOWING | OBSESSIVE BEHAVIOUR | | IMPAIRED VOLUNTARY MOVEMENTS | DIFFICULTY CONCENTRATING | IRRITABILITY | IMPULSIVENESS | DEPRESSION | | APATHY | ANGER | LACK OF EMOTION | PERIODS OF AGGRESSION | PERIODS OF EXCITEMENT | EMOTIONAL ISSUES | | INSOMNIA | FATIGUE | OTHER:			
	6. Highlight any activities of daily living which are affected by Huntington's disease: | GETTING UP FROM A CHAIR | | RISING FROM BED | GOING TO BED WASHING | DRESSING | UNDRESSING | CUTTING FOOD UP | EATING | DRINKING | | GOING TO THE TOILET | MOBILISING | ATTENDING ACTIVITIES |			
	7. Note in detail the daily routine and the agreed assistance required by the patient for the activities of daily living:			

Copyright © 2020 Planning For Care Limited

CARE PLAN: Huntington's Disease

This care plan must be reviewed monthly (or more often if required) and each action must be signed and dated

Patient's Issues and Objectives	Consultation Assessment and Plan	Signature	Date	Review Date
	8. Note the agreed plan of care for the patient's mobility and periods of rest to prevent fatigue:			
	9. Highlight any specialised equipment that may assist the patient: | ANTI SPILLAGE CUP | ADAPTED CUTLERY | MECHANICAL HELPING HAND | NONSLIP MATS | PLATE GUARDS |			
	10. Note the prescribed medication, dose and frequency:			
	11. Monitor the patient's nutritional state and weight monthly or more frequently if required.			
	12. Liaise with the General Practitioner as necessary.			

Name	Patient/Relative Signature	Date

Copyright © 2020 Planning For Care Limited

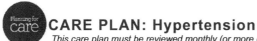

CARE PLAN: Hypertension

This care plan must be reviewed monthly (or more often if required) and each action must be signed and dated

High blood pressure or hypertension means a high pressure in the arteries. Arteries are vessels that carry blood from the pumping heart to all the tissues and organs of the body. Normal blood pressure is below 120/80, blood pressure of 140/90 or above is considered high. The higher number, the systolic blood pressure is the pressure in the arteries as the heart contracts and pumps blood forward into the arteries. The lower number, the diastolic pressure is the pressure in the arteries as the heart relaxes after the contraction. Hypertension can lead to a heart attack, heart failure, stroke, dementia, or kidney disease but the condition hardly ever shows any signs and symptoms and can go undetected.

Patient's Issues and Objectives	Consultation Assessment and Plan	Signature	Date	Review Date
Hypertension To maintain blood pressure within normal limits	1. Discuss the condition with the patient and, or relative and agree the plan of care.			
	2. Note the patient's and, or relative's understanding of the condition and any concerns or anxieties they have:			
	3. Note the past history of hypertension, any symptoms experienced, and treatment received:			
	4. Highlight any of the following symptoms experienced by the patient: | HEADACHE | BLURRED VISION | DOUBLE VISION | NOSE BLEEDS | SHORTNESS OF BREATH |			
	5. Note the patient's blood pressure and pulse:			
	6. Highlight any contributing factors: | OBESITY | SMOKING | DIABETES TYPE I | DIABETES TYPE 2 | KIDNEY DISEASE | EXCESSIVE ALCOHOL | | EXCESSIVE SALT | LACK OF EXERCISE | MEDICATION, STEROIDS |................			
	7. Note any agreed plan for lifestyle changes where appropriate:			
	8. Note the prescribed anti hypertensive medication, dose and frequency:			
	9. Note the General Practitioner's instructions for monitoring blood pressure and frequency:			

Copyright © 2020 Planning For Care Limited

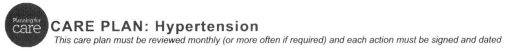
CARE PLAN: Hypertension

This care plan must be reviewed monthly (or more often if required) and each action must be signed and dated

Patient's Issues and Objectives	Consultation Assessment and Plan	Signature	Date	Review Date
	10. Monitor and document any symptoms of severe hypertension such as headaches, sleepiness or confusion.			
	11. Liaise with the General Practitioner as required.			

Name	Patient/Relative Signature	Date

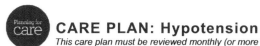

CARE PLAN: Hypotension

This care plan must be reviewed monthly (or more often if required) and each action must be signed and dated

Low blood pressure or hypotension means a low pressure in the arteries. Arteries are vessels, which carry blood from the pumping heart to all the tissues and organs of the body. Normal blood pressure is approximately 120/80, blood pressure of 90/60 or below is considered low. The higher number, the systolic blood pressure is the pressure in the arteries as the heart contracts and pumps blood forward into the arteries. The lower number, the diastolic pressure is the pressure in the arteries as the heart relaxes after the contraction. When the flow of blood is too low to deliver enough oxygen and nutrients to vital organs such as the brain, heart, and kidney, the organs do not function normally and may be temporarily or permanently damaged. Hypotension can cause fainting or feeling dizzy but the condition hardly ever shows any signs and symptoms and can go undetected. Naturally low blood pressure does not usually need to be treated unless it is causing symptoms such as dizziness, unsteadiness, fainting, or recurrent falls.

Patient's Issues and Objectives	Consultation Assessment and Plan	Signature	Date	Review Date
Hypotension To manage and minimise the symptoms of hypotension	1. Discuss the condition with the patient and, or relative and agree the plan of care.			
	2. Note the patient's and, or relative's understanding of the condition and any concerns or anxieties they have:			
	3. Note the past history of hypotension and any symptoms experienced:			
	4. Note the patient's blood pressure: Sitting BP.................... Standing BP....................			
	5. Highlight the symptoms experienced by the patient: | LIGHTHEADED | DIZZY | RECURRENT FALLS | DIZZY WHEN STANDING FROM A SITTING OR LYING POSITION | | FAINTING | UNSTEADINESS |............			
	6. Highlight the agreed plan of care to minimise the effects of low blood pressure: • To stand up gradually • To wear support stockings • To avoid caffeine at night and limit alcohol intake • To include more salt in the diet • To eat smaller meals, more often			

Copyright © 2020 Planning For Care Limited

CARE PLAN: Hypotension

This care plan must be reviewed monthly (or more often if required) and each action must be signed and dated

Patient's Issues and Objectives	Consultation Assessment and Plan	Signature	Date	Review Date
	7. If the patient is a high risk of falling at night, note the agreed safety measures to minimise the risk:			
	8. Note the General Practitioner's instructions for monitoring blood pressure and frequency:			
	9. Liaise with the General Practitioner as required.			
	....			

Name	Patient/Relative Signature	Date

CARE PLAN Implantable Cardioverter Defibrillator:
This care plan must be reviewed monthly (or more often if required) and each action must be signed and dated

An implantable cardioverter-defibrillator, ICD, is a small device, similar to a pacemaker, which is surgically placed under the skin, usually below the left collarbone. One or two, insulated wires run from the ICD through veins to the lower chambers of the heart. It detects and stops abnormal heartbeats, or arrhythmias. It continuously monitors the heartbeat and delivers extra beats or electrical shocks to restore a normal heart rhythm, when necessary. An ICD differs from a pacemaker, which can be used to treat less dangerous heart rhythms, such as those that occur in the upper chambers of the heart. The ICD can be programmed for low-energy pacing therapy, which responds to mild disruptions in heartbeat, cardioversion therapy where a higher energy shock is delivered to deal with a more serious heart rhythm problem, or defibrillation therapy which is the strongest form of electrical therapy used to restore a normal heartbeat. Usually, only one shock is needed to restore a normal heartbeat. However, sometimes two or more such shocks are required during a 24-hour period. Frequent shocks in a short time are known as an ICD storm, which is a medical emergency. The ICD must be checked to see if it is working properly or if there is a problem that is making the heart beat more abnormally. If necessary, the ICD can be adjusted to reduce the number and frequency of shocks. Additional medications may be required to ensure the heart beats regularly and decreases the chance of an ICD storm.

Patient's Issues and Objectives	Consultation Assessment and Plan	Signature	Date	Review Date
Implantable cardioverter-defibrillator To monitor the effects of the implantable cardioverter-defibrillator To maintain an optimum level of health	**1. Discuss the implantable cardioverter-defibrillator, ICD with the patient and, or relative and agree the plan of care.**			
	2. Note the patient's and, or relative's understanding of the ICD and any concerns or anxieties they have:			
	3. Highlight the reason for the implantable cardioverter-defibrillator: | CORONARY ARTERY DISEASE AND HEART ATTACK | INHERITED HEART DEFECT | VENTRICULAR TACHYCARDIA | | VENTRICULAR FIBRILLATION | CARDIOMYOPATHY OR THICKENED HEART MUSCLE | OTHER:............................			
	4. Note the patient's past history of cardiac disease, symptoms experienced, and any treatment received:			
	5. Note the patient's baseline temperature pulse, respirations and blood pressure:			
	6. Note when the implantable cardioverter-defibrillator was fitted:			
	7. Note how frequently the clinic requires to check the implantable cardioverter-defibrillator. The lithium battery in the ICD can last up to 7 years but must it be checked every 3-6 months:			
	8. Discuss the importance of informing all doctors, dentists, and medical technicians of the ICD as some medical procedures can disrupt the ICD, such as magnetic resonance imaging, MRI, magnetic resonance angiography, MRA, and radiofrequency or microwave ablation.			

Copyright © 2020 Planning For Care Limited

CARE PLAN Implantable Cardioverter Defibrillator:
This care plan must be reviewed monthly (or more often if required) and each action must be signed and dated

Patient's Issues and Objectives	Consultation Assessment and Plan	Signature	Date	Review Date
	9. Explain that microwave ovens, televisions, remote controls, radios, toasters, electric blankets, electric shavers, electric drills, computers, scanners, printers, and GPS devices pose little or no risk to the functioning of the ICD.			
	10. Discuss the importance of avoiding close or prolonged contact with devices which have strong magnetic fields as these can disrupt the electrical signalling of the cardioverter-defibrillator and stop it from working. • Cell phones and other mobile devices should be kept 15cms from the ICD site • The ICD may set off airport security alarms or other security systems • Hand-held metal detectors often contain a magnet that may interfere with the ICD • Power generators, welding equipment, high-voltage transformers or motor-generator systems can affect an ICD • MP3 player headphones contain a magnetic substance and can interfere with the ICD			
	11. Contact the General Practitioner immediately if there are any signs that the ICD is not functioning properly.			
	....			

Name	Patient/Relative Signature	Date

Copyright © 2020 Planning For Care Limited

CARE PLAN: Irritable Bowel Syndrome

This care plan must be reviewed monthly (or more often if required) and each action must be signed and dated

Irritable bowel syndrome, IBS, is a common, long-term condition of the digestive system. Irritable bowel syndrome is characterised by increased or decreased strength and duration of intestinal contractions. Increased contractions cause the contents to move through the intestinal tract too quickly, whereas decreased contractions causes intestinal contents to remain stagnant in the bowel. Symptoms of irritable bowel syndrome include loose stools, bloating, gas, mucous, in the stool, constipation, abdominal cramps and the strong urge to have a bowel movement. Irritable bowel syndrome can usually be managed by following a balanced diet and the avoidance of trigger foods. Although every case is different, common trigger foods include alcohol, fizzy drinks, chocolate, dairy products, beans, caffeine, fatty foods and processed snacks such as crisps and biscuits.

Patient's Issues and Objectives	Consultation Assessment and Plan	Signature	Date	Review Date
Irritable Bowel Syndrome **To regain normal bowel function and promote effective management**	1. Discuss the condition with the patient and, or relative and agree the plan of care.			
	2. Note the patient's and, or relative's understanding of the condition and any concerns or anxieties they have:			
	3. Note the past medical history of the bowel condition, when it was diagnosed, any treatment prescribed and how effective it was:			
	4. Highlight any signs and symptoms experienced by the patient: | ABDOMINAL PAIN | DIARRHOEA | CONSTIPATION | BLOATING | FLATULENCE | MUCOUS IN FAECES | NAUSEA | | URGENT NEED TO GO TO HAVE A BOWEL MOVEMENT | FEELING THAT THE BOWELS ARE NOT FULLY EMPTY | | LETHARGY | FATIGUE | BACKACHE | BLADDER PROBLEMS URGENT NEED TO URINATE | FAECAL INCONTINENCE |			
	5. Highlight any known triggers: | STRESS | ALCOHOL | BUTTER | MAYONNAISE | MARGARINE AND OIL | CARBONATED DRINKS | COFFEE | TEA | | CHOCOLATE | CORN | DAIRY PRODUCTS | FATTY FRIED FOODS | FOODS HIGH IN FIBRE | BROCCOLI | LENTILS | | GAS PRODUCING FOODS | BEANS | CABBAGE | ONIONS | NUTS AND SEEDS | PEANUT BUTTER | WHOLE GRAINS | | BRAN | RAW VEGETABLES | RAW FRUITS | RED MEAT AND PORK | SPICY FOODS |			
	6. Agree with the patient and, or relatives the diet plan and note any issues the patient may have avoiding the trigger foods, due to memory or other issues:			

Copyright © 2020 Planning For Care Limited

CARE PLAN: Irritable Bowel Syndrome

This care plan must be reviewed monthly (or more often if required) and each action must be signed and dated

Patient's Issues and Objectives	Consultation Assessment and Plan	Signature	Date	Review Date
	7. Note the patient's normal bowel function: Frequency.. Time of day..			
	8. Note the prescribed medication, dose and frequency:			
	9. Encourage sufficient fluid intake 1500mls - 2000mls per day.			
	10. Note if there are any issues the patient has drinking adequate fluids and the agreed care plan to improve this:			
	11. Liaise with the patient's General Practitioner, as necessary.			

Name	Patient/Relative Signature	Date

Copyright © 2020 Planning For Care Limited

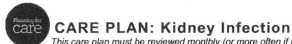

CARE PLAN: Kidney Infection

This care plan must be reviewed monthly (or more often if required) and each action must be signed and dated

A kidney infection is a painful and unpleasant infection, which usually happens when bacteria travel from the bladder into one or both of the kidneys. A kidney infection requires prompt treatment because as it develops it can cause permanent kidney damage. Often the symptoms manifest themselves quickly, within a few hours, and they can cause fever, shivering, nausea, sickness, and lower back pain. Most kidney infections need prompt treatment with antibiotics to stop the infection from damaging the kidneys or spreading to the bloodstream. As this can be a very painful infection painkillers may be prescribed.

Patient's Issues and Objectives	Consultation Assessment and Plan	Signature	Date	Review Date
Kidney Infection To effectively treat the infection, promote recovery and reduce the risk of the infection re-occurring	1. Discuss the condition with the patient and, or relatives and agree the plan of care.			
	2. Note the patient's and, or relative's understanding of the condition and any concerns or anxieties they have:			
	3. Note any past history of kidney infections, the frequency and treatment:			
	4. Highlight which of the following signs and symptoms the patient is experiencing: | FREQUENTLY FEELING THE NEED TO URINATE | FREQUENTLY NEEDING TO URINATE | FOUL SMELLING URINE | | UNABLE TO URINATE FULLY | CLOUDY URINE | BLOOD IN URINE | FEVER | UNCHARACTERISTIC CONFUSION | | INCREASED CONFUSION | SHIVERING | NAUSEA | SICKNESS | FATIGUE | PAIN WHEN URINATING | ACUTE PAIN | | LOWER BACK PAIN | PAIN IN GENITAL AREA | LOSS OF APPETITE | DIARRHOEA |............			
	5. Highlight any contributing factors: | URINARY INCONTINENCE | URINARY RETENTION | CATHETER | DIABETES | | PROSTATE ENLARGEMENT | PROLAPSE OF THE PELVIC ORGANS | URINARY TRACT INFECTION | | RECURRENT URINARY TRACT INFECTIONS | KIDNEY STONES |............			
	6. Consult the patient's General Practitioner and detail advice given:			
	7. Note the prescribed medication, dose and frequency:			
	8. Discuss the importance of taking an adequate fluid intake 1500-2000mls daily and encourage this.			
	9. Where the patient's fluid intake is inadequate, specify the plan of care to improve the intake and commence a fluid balance chart:............			

Copyright © 2020 Planning For Care Limited

CARE PLAN: Kidney Infection

This care plan must be reviewed monthly (or more often if required) and each action must be signed and dated

Patient's Issues and Objectives	Consultation Assessment and Plan	Signature	Date	Review Date
	10. Note the patient's preferences for fluids:			
	11. Four days after the completion of the course of antibiotics a further MSSU must be sent to the laboratory and the results must be recorded in the patient's notes.			
	12. Liaise with the General Practitioner as necessary.			

Name	Patient/Relative Signature	Date

CARE PLAN: Korsakoff's Syndrome

This care plan must be reviewed monthly (or more often if required) and each action must be signed and dated

Wernicke Korsakoff's Syndrome, commonly known as Korsakoff's Syndrome, is a brain disorder usually caused by heavy alcohol consumption over a long period. Although it is not strictly speaking a dementia, people with the condition experience loss of short-term memory. It is caused by lack of thiamine, vitamin B1, which affects the brain and nervous system. People who drink alcohol excessively are often thiamine deficient, because their diet is poor and does not contain vitamins. Alcohol can interfere with the conversion of thiamine into the active form of the vitamin B1. It can inflame the stomach lining, cause vomiting and make it difficult for the body to absorb vitamins. Alcohol also makes it harder for the liver to store vitamins. The main symptom is memory loss, particularly of events that occur after the onset of the condition. Other symptoms may include difficulty in retaining new information or learning new skills, lack of insight, confabulation, where a person invents events to fill the gaps in memory, change in personality, at one extreme, lack of emotional reaction, or at the other, being talkative and repetitive. Unlike Alzheimer's disease or vascular dementia, Korsakoff's syndrome is not certain to get worse over time. It can be halted if the person is given high doses of thiamine, abstains from alcohol, and adopts a healthy diet with vitamin supplements.

Patient's Issues and Objectives	Consultation Assessment and Plan	Signature	Date	Review Date
Korsakoff's Syndrome To maintain an optimal level of independence and quality of life	1. Discuss the condition with the patient and, or relative and agree the plan of care.			
	2. Note the patient's and, or relative's understanding of the condition and any concerns or anxieties they have:			
	3. Ensure the Life Story Book and a day in the life of the patient is completed and incorporated into this Care Plan.			
	4. Note when the patient was diagnosed and outline the past history:			
	5. Highlight the symptoms experienced by the patient: | MALNOURISHED | INVOLUNTARY EYE MOVEMENTS | JERKY EYE MOVEMENTS | PARALYSIS OF EYE MUSCLES | | POOR BALANCE | UNSTEADINESS | DISORIENTATED | CONFUSED | MILD MEMORY LOSS | CONFABULATION | OTHER:			
	6. Specify any issues the patient has with communication and the agreed plan to address these:			
	7. Note any emotional or anxiety issues the patient has, how they are manifest, and the agreed plan to address these:			
	8. Highlight any of the activities of daily living, the patient has issues with, or needs assistance with: | RISING FROM BED | GOING TO BED | USING WALKING AIDS | WALKING | MOBILISING | WASHING | DRESSING | | UNDRESSING | CUTTING FOOD UP | EATING | DRINKING | GOING TO THE TOILET | ATTENDING ACTIVITIES |			

Copyright © 2020 Planning For Care Limited

CARE PLAN: Korsakoff's Syndrome

This care plan must be reviewed monthly (or more often if required) and each action must be signed and dated

Patient's Issues and Objectives	Consultation Assessment and Plan	Signature	Date	Review Date
	9. Note in detail the agreed plan of care to assist the patient with the activities they have issues with:			
	10. Specify any issues the patient has with regards to safety, any associated risks and the agreed plan to address these:			
	11. Note the prescribed medication, the dose and frequency:			
	12. Liaise with the General Practitioner and, or Psychogeriatrician as required.			

Name	Patient/Relative Signature	Date

Copyright © 2020 Planning For Care Limited

CARE PLAN: Labyrinthitis Inner Ear Infection

This care plan must be reviewed monthly (or more often if required) and each action must be signed and dated

Labyrinthitis is an inner ear infection. It causes a delicate structure deep inside the ear called the labyrinth to become inflamed, affecting hearing and balance. The labyrinth is the innermost part of the ear. It usually becomes inflamed either because of a viral infection, such as a cold or flu or a bacterial infection, which is much less common. The most common symptoms are dizziness, hearing loss, from mild to total loss of hearing, and vertigo, the sensation that you, or the environment around you, is moving. In most cases, the symptoms pass within a few weeks. Treatment involves a combination of bed rest and medication to help with the symptoms. Additional medication may be needed to fight the underlying infection, although antibiotics are not often required as the cause is most commonly due to a virus. Labyrinthitis often develops in people who have an underlying autoimmune condition, where the immune system mistakenly attacks healthy tissue rather than fighting off infections.

Patient's Issues and Objectives	Consultation Assessment and Plan	Signature	Date	Review Date
Labyrinthitis Inner Ear Infection To relieve any associated symptoms and effectively treat the infection	1. Discuss the condition with the patient and, or relative and agree the plan of care.			
	2. Note the patient's and, or relative's understanding of the issue and any concerns or anxieties they have:			
	3. Note the patient's past history of ear infections:			
	4. Which ear is affected:	LEFT	RIGHT	BOTH				
	5. Highlight the symptoms evident or experienced by the patient:	DIZZINESS	MILD HEARING LOSS	SEVERE HEARING LOSS	VERTIGO	A FEELING OF PRESSURE INSIDE THE EAR		RINGING	HUMMING	TINNITUS	FLUID DISCHARGE	PUS DISCHARGE	EAR ACHE	MILD HEADACHE	NAUSEA		VOMITING	FEVER	BLURRED VISION	DOUBLE VISION	HIGH TEMPERATURE |....................................			
	6. Consult the General Practitioner for advice and detail any prescribed medication:			
	7. Highlight anything that makes the feeling of dizziness worse for the patient:	THE DARK	BEING IN A CROWDED AREA	TIREDNESS	WALKING	HEIGHTS	MENSTRUAL CYCLE	....			
	8. Discuss with the patient and or relative and highlight the agreed plan of care to alleviate or address the symptoms:	LIE DOWN ON ONE SIDE DURING A VERTIGO ATTACK	AVOID ALCOHOL	AVOID BRIGHT LIGHTS	CUT OUT NOISE	....			

Copyright © 2020 Planning For Care Limited

CARE PLAN: Labyrinthitis Inner Ear Infection

This care plan must be reviewed monthly (or more often if required) and each action must be signed and dated

Patient's Issues and Objectives	Consultation Assessment and Plan	Signature	Date	Review Date
	9. If the patient is a high risk of falling at night, detail any agreed safety measures to be put in place:			
	10. Monitor the patient's condition and liaise with the General Practitioner as necessary.			

Name	Patient/Relative Signature	Date

Copyright © 2020 Planning For Care Limited

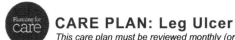

CARE PLAN: Leg Ulcer

This care plan must be reviewed monthly (or more often if required) and each action must be signed and dated

A leg ulcer is a chronic, long lasting, wound on the leg or foot that takes longer than six weeks to heal. Leg ulcers affect the lower limbs and can be mainly venous, arterial or neuropathic. A venous leg ulcer can develop after a minor injury if there is a problem with the circulation of blood in the veins of the leg. If this happens, the pressure inside the veins increases. This constant high pressure can gradually damage the tiny blood vessels in your skin and make it fragile. As a result, the skin can easily break and form an ulcer after a knock or scratch.

Patient's Issues and Objectives	Consultation Assessment and Plan	Signature	Date	Review Date
Leg Ulcer	1. Discuss the condition with the patient and, or relative and agree the plan of care.			
	2. Note the patient's and, or the relative's understanding of the condition and any concerns or anxieties they have:			
To heal the leg ulcer	3. Identify the area(s) affected:			
Promotion and maintenance of healthy skin	4. Discuss with the patient and, or relative any possible contributing factors and highlight them: | POOR CIRCULATION | DIABETES | SMOKING | HIGH BLOOD PRESSURE | ARTHRITIS | HEART DISEASE | OBESITY | | ATHEROSCLEROSIS IN THE LEGS |............			
	5. Note the agreed plan to improve the contributing factors, where possible:			
	6. Highlight any associated or other symptoms experienced by the patient: | SWOLLEN ANKLES | SWOLLEN LEGS | DISCOLOURATION AND DARKENING OF THE SKIN AROUND THE ULCER | | ACHING LEGS | HEAVY FEELING IN LEGS | HARDENED SKIN AROUND ULCER | FLAKY SCALEY SKIN ON LEGS | | SWOLLEN AND ENLARGED VEINS ON LEGS | FOUL SMELLING DISCHARGE |............			
	7. Consult with the patient's General Practitioner			
	8. Note the prescribed medication and treatment regime:			

Copyright © 2020 Planning For Care Limited

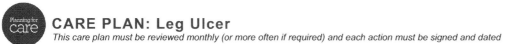

CARE PLAN: Leg Ulcer

This care plan must be reviewed monthly (or more often if required) and each action must be signed and dated

Patient's Issues and Objectives	Consultation Assessment and Plan	Signature	Date	Review Date
	9. Highlight any additional agreed plan of care to promote healing: • compression bandage • elevate legs, feet at a higher position than the heart when sitting • avoid standing for long periods • moderate exercise • moisturise dry flaky skin			
	10. Complete wound assessment chart and update as necessary.			
	11. Liaise with the patient's General Practitioner as required.			

Name	Patient/Relative Signature	Date

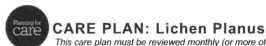

CARE PLAN: Lichen Planus

This care plan must be reviewed monthly (or more often if required) and each action must be signed and dated

Lichen planus is a non-infectious, itchy rash that can affect many areas of the body. The symptoms of lichen planus of the skin are purple-red coloured bumps, papules, which are slightly raised, shiny and have a flat top. The papules usually measure 3-5mm in diameter and may also have irregular white streaks, Wickham's striae, thicker scaly patches can appear, usually around the ankles, this is known as hypertrophic lichen planus. Lichen planus of the skin often affects the wrists, ankles and lower back, although other parts of the body can also be affected. Thickened hypertrophic lichen planus affects the shins, and ring-shaped lichen planus affects creases in the skin, such as the armpits, mouth, penis, vulva or vagina. After the papules have cleared, the affected area of skin can sometimes become discoloured. Lichen planus is thought to be caused by the immune system, or an abnormal response of the immune system to certain medicines. There's no single treatment that can cure lichen planus completely. However, treatments such as steroid creams or ointments are available to help relieve the itch and control the rash and make living with it easier.

Patient's Issues and Objectives	Consultation Assessment and Plan	Signature	Date	Review Date
Lichen Planus **Promotion and maintenance of healthy skin**	1. Discuss the condition with the patient and, or relative and agree the plan of care.			
	2. Note the patient's and, or the relative's understanding of the condition and any concerns or anxieties they have:			
	3. Note the past history of the condition and the treatment received:			
	4. Note the cause if known:			
	5. Identify the area(s) of the body affected by Lichen Planus:			
	6. Highlight the signs and symptoms experienced by the patient: • purple-red coloured bumps, papules, which are slightly raised, shiny and have a flat top, usually 3-5mm in diameter and may also have irregular white streaks, Wickham's striae • thicker scaly patches can appear, usually around the ankles – this is known as hypertrophic lichen planus • itchy skin			
	7. Note the prescribed treatment:			

Copyright © 2020 Planning For Care Limited

CARE PLAN: Lichen Planus

This care plan must be reviewed monthly (or more often if required) and each action must be signed and dated

Patient's Issues and Objectives	Consultation Assessment and Plan	Signature	Date	Review Date
	8. Highlight the agreed plan of care: | AVOID WASHING WITH SOAP | USE ONLY WATER TO WASH | USE EMOLLIENT TO MOISTURISE SKIN | | WHEN WASHING HAIR AVOID SHAMPOO COMING INTO CONTACT WITH AFFECTED AREAS OF SKIN |			
	9. Identify any issues the patient may have with the application of creams:			
	10. Monitor the patient's condition and liaise with the General Practitioner as necessary.			

Name	Patient/Relative Signature	Date

Copyright © 2020 Planning For Care Limited

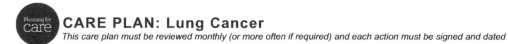

CARE PLAN: Lung Cancer

This care plan must be reviewed monthly (or more often if required) and each action must be signed and dated

Lung cancer is one of the most common and serious types of cancer, characterised by uncontrolled cell growth in cells of the lung. Cancer that begins in the lungs is called primary lung cancer. Cancer that spreads to the lungs from another place in the body is known as secondary lung cancer. There are two main types of primary lung cancer, non-small-cell lung cancer, the most common type, which can be either, squamous cell carcinoma, adenocarcinoma or large-cell carcinoma, and small-cell lung cancer, which can be faster spreading. The type of treatment depends on the type of cancer, and how far the cancer has spread. If the condition is diagnosed early and the cancerous cells are confined to a small area, surgery to remove the affected area of lung is usually recommended. Breathlessness is common in people with lung cancer, whether it is a symptom of the condition or a side effect of treatment.

Patient's Issues and Objectives	Consultation Assessment and Plan	Signature	Date	Review Date
Lung Cancer **To promote ease of breathing** **To maintain an optimal level of independence and lifestyle**	1. Discuss the condition with the patient and, or relative and agree the plan of care.			
	2. Note the patient's and, or relative's understanding of the cancer and any concerns or anxieties they have:			
	3. Highlight the cause of the lung cancer if known: | SMOKING | PASSIVE SMOKING | EXPOSURE TO CHEMICALS | | POLLUTION |..			
	4. Highlight the diagnosed stage of the lung cancer, where known: • Stage I. Early cancer that is confined to the lung, and the tumour is smaller than 5cms • Stage II. The tumour may have grown larger than 5cms, or it may be a small tumour that involves nearby structures such as the chest wall, diaphragm, or the lining of the lungs, the pleura, and may have spread to the lymph nodes • Stage III. The tumour may have grown very large and invaded other organs near the lungs. This stage may indicate a smaller tumour with cancer cells in lymph nodes further away from the lungs • Stage IV. The Cancer has spread beyond the affected lung to the other lung or to distant areas of the body			
	5. Note the past history of lung cancer and any respiratory issues and treatments prescribed or received:			
	6. Highlight the symptoms experienced by the patient: | PERSISTENT COUGH | PERSISTENT CHEST INFECTIONS | | COUGHING UP BLOOD | TIREDNESS | WEIGHT LOSS | PERSISTENT BREATHLESSNESS | ACHE WHEN BREATHING | | PAIN WHEN BREATHING | FINGER CLUBBING | HIGH TEMPERATURE | DIFFICULTY SWALLOWING | SWOLLEN FACE | | SWOLLEN NECK | WHEEZING | PAIN WHEN SWALLOWING | PERSISTENT CHEST PAIN | PERSISTENT SHOULDER PAIN |			

CARE PLAN: Lung Cancer

This care plan must be reviewed monthly (or more often if required) and each action must be signed and dated

Patient's Issues and Objectives	Consultation Assessment and Plan	Signature	Date	Review Date
	7. Note the prescribed medication, dose and frequency if applicable: 			
	8. Detail the living conditions the patient prefers to help them psychologically or physically: Ventilation: .... Fans: .... Room temperature: .... Number of pillows required: .... Preferred position whilst in bed:			
	9. Detail any of the activities of daily living with which, the patient has issues: 			
	10. Note the agreed plan of care to address the issues the patient has with any of the activities of daily living: 			
	11. Monitor the patient's condition and liaise with the General Practitioner or Consultant as required. 			

Name	Patient/Relative Signature	Date

Copyright © 2020 Planning For Care Limited

CARE PLAN: Medication Administration

This care plan must be reviewed monthly (or more often if required) and each action must be signed and dated

In order to get the maximum benefit from medications, it is important that all medication is taken exactly as prescribed by the doctor. All medicines must be administered at the prescribed time, in the correct dose and in accordance with the prescribed route of administration. Nurses and carers may be responsible for administering medications and they must be knowledgeable about the effects, side effects and interactions of medications and take action as necessary. It is not solely a mechanistic task to be performed in strict compliance with the written prescription of a medical practitioner, it requires thought and the exercise of professional judgement.

Patient's Issues and Objectives	Consultation Assessment and Plan	Signature	Date	Review Date
Taking the correct prescribed medication at the prescribed times **To assist the patient with the administration of the correct medication and dose at the prescribed times.**	1. Discuss with the patient and, or relatives any issues the patient has taking or receiving their prescribed medication or treatment.			
	2. Note the patient and, or relatives understanding of the issues and any anxieties or concerns they may have:			
	3. Highlight any physical or mental issues the patient may have with regards to taking medication: | SWALLOWING ISSUES REQUIRING ADDITION OF THICKENER TO FLUIDS | POOR EYESIGHT | REGISTERED BLIND | | SWALLOWING ISSUES NEEDING LOTS OF FLUID | MENTAL HEALTH ISSUES | LACK OF UNDERSTANDING | | PARANOIA, BELIEF THAT THE MEDICATION IS NOT GOOD | PHYSICAL DISABILITY | SPECIFY:.................			
	4. Specify the patient's issue or issues taking oral medication, or having instilled prescribed medication, or topically applied medication:			
	5. Note if the patient's issues regarding medication varies from day to day and how this can manifest:			
	6. Note in detail the agreed plan of care to assist the patient to take the prescribed medication:			

Copyright © 2020 Planning For Care Limited

CARE PLAN: Medication Administration

This care plan must be reviewed monthly (or more often if required) and each action must be signed and dated

Patient's Issues and Objectives	Consultation Assessment and Plan	Signature	Date	Review Date
	7. Record in detail if the patient is unable to take or refuses to take the prescribed medication.			
	8. Liaise with the patient's General Practitioner as necessary.			

Name	Patient/Relative Signature	Date

Copyright © 2020 Planning For Care Limited

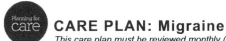

CARE PLAN: Migraine
This care plan must be reviewed monthly (or more often if required) and each action must be signed and dated

A migraine is usually a severe headache felt as a throbbing pain at the front or side of the head. Some people may also have other symptoms, such as nausea, vomiting or increased sensitivity to light or sound. They usually begin in early adulthood. There are several types, including a migraine with aura, where there are warning signs before the migraine begins, such as seeing flashing lights, a migraine without aura where it occurs without warning signs, a migraine aura without headache, also known as silent migraine, where an aura or other migraine symptoms are experienced, but a headache does not develop. Some people have migraines frequently, up to several times a week, others only have a migraine occasionally. Migraine attacks can be associated with certain triggers, which can include stress, tiredness and certain foods or drinks. It is important to seek medical advice if, a migraine lasts for more than 72 hours. This type of migraine is known as status migrainosus.

Patient's Issues and Objectives	Consultation Assessment and Plan	Signature	Date	Review Date
Migraine To alleviate pain, promote comfort and alleviate associated issues	1. Discuss the issue with the patient and, or relative and agree the plan of care.			
	2. Note any previous medical history of migraine and the treatment prescribed:			
	3. Highlight any specific trigger for a migraine: | STRESS | CHANGES IN SLEEP PATTERN | TENSION IN NECK | CHOCOLATE | SKIPPING MEALS CHEESE | ALCOHOL | | CAFFEINE | STRENUOUS EXERCISE WHEN NOT USED TO IT | LOUD NOISES | BRIGHT LIGHT | FLICKERING LIGHTS | | NOT DRINKING ENOUGH FLUID | HORMONAL | EMOTIONAL | MEDICINAL | ENVIRONMENTAL |...........................			
	4. Highlight any warning signs the patient has: | VISUAL PROBLEMS | FLASHIING LIGHTS | VISUAL BLIND SPOTS | | FEELS DIZZY | DIFFICULTY SPEAKING | TINGLING |...........................			
	5. Highlight any symptoms experienced: | HEADACHE | NAUSEA | VOMITING | INCREASED SENSITVITY TO LIGHT | | SWEATING | POOR CONCENTRATION | ABDOMINAL PAIN | DIARRHOEA | SPECIFY:			
	6. Consult with the patient's General Practitioner and note the prescribed medication, dose and frequency:			
	7. Detail the agreed plan of care:			

Copyright © 2020 Planning For Care Limited

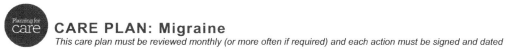

CARE PLAN: Migraine

This care plan must be reviewed monthly (or more often if required) and each action must be signed and dated

Patient's Issues and Objectives	Consultation Assessment and Plan	Signature	Date	Review Date
	8. Consult the General Practitioner immediately, if the patient shows any signs of the following: • paralysis or weakness in one or both arms and, or one side of the face • slurred or garbled speech • a sudden agonising headache resulting in a blinding pain unlike anything experienced before • headache along with a high temperature (fever), stiff neck, mental confusion, seizures, double vision, and a rash			
	9. Monitor effectiveness of treatment and where necessary liaise with the patient's General Practitioner.			

Name	Patient/Relative Signature	Date

CARE PLAN: Mild Cognitive Impairment

This care plan must be reviewed monthly (or more often if required) and each action must be signed and dated

Mild cognitive impairment, MCI, is a condition where there are minor problems with cognition, or mental abilities such as memory or thinking. In MCI these difficulties are worse than would normally be expected for a healthy person of the same age. However, the symptoms are not severe enough to interfere significantly with daily life, and so are not defined as dementia. A person with MCI has mild problems with, memory, or reasoning, planning or problem-solving, or attention, being easily distracted, or taking much longer to find the right word for something, or visual depth, struggling to judge distances or navigate stairs. People with MCI are at increased risk of deteriorating to greater levels of impairment and dementia. However, this is not true of all. It is currently difficult to determine in advance who will regress or deteriorate and those who will not.

Patient's Issues and Objectives	Consultation Assessment and Plan	Signature	Date	Review Date
Mild Cognitive Impairment To maintain an optimal level of independence and quality of life	1. Discuss the condition with the patient and, or relative and agree the plan of care.			
	2. Note the patient's and, or the relative's understanding of the condition and any concerns or anxieties they have:			
	3. Ensure the Life Story Book and a day in the life of the patient is completed and incorporated into this Care Plan.			
	4. Note when the patient was diagnosed and outline the past history:			
	5. Highlight any signs and symptoms experienced by the patient: • memory, forgetting recent events or repeating the same question • reasoning, planning or problem-solving, struggling with thinking things through • attention, being very easily distracted • language, taking much longer than usual to find the right word for something • visual depth perception, struggling to interpret an object in three dimensions, judge distances or navigate stairs.			
	6. Specify the type of memory issues that the patient experiences:			
	7. Specify any issues the patient has with communication and the agreed plan to address them:			
	8. Specify any issues the patient has with regards to safety, the risks, and the agreed plan to address them:			

Copyright © 2020 Planning For Care Limited

CARE PLAN: Mild Cognitive Impairment

This care plan must be reviewed monthly (or more often if required) and each action must be signed and dated

Patient's Issues and Objectives	Consultation Assessment and Plan	Signature	Date	Review Date
	9. Highlight any of the following activities the patient has issues with, or needs assistance with: | RISING FROM BED | GOING TO BED | USING WALKING AIDS | WALKING | MOBILISING | WASHING | DRESSING | | UNDRESSING | CUTTING FOOD UP | EATING | DRINKING | GOING TO THE TOILET | ATTENDING ACTIVITIES | OTHER:			
	10. Note in detail the agreed plan of care for any of the activities of living, that the patient has issues with:			
	11. Note any emotional or anxiety issues the patient has, how they are manifest, and the agreed plan to address them:			
	12. Note the prescribed medication, the dose, and frequency:			
	13. Liaise with the General Practitioner as required.			

Name	Patient/Relative Signature	Date

Copyright © 2020 Planning For Care Limited

CARE PLAN: Mobility and Physical Activity

This care plan must be reviewed monthly (or more often if required) and each action must be signed and dated

Mobility and physical activity, such as regular exercise, is important for health. People who are chronically ill, elderly, or disabled are particularly susceptible to the adverse effects of prolonged bed rest, immobilisation, and inactivity. The effects of immobility are rarely confined to only one body system. Immobility may later cause a wide range of complications. Immobility in the elderly often cannot be prevented, but many of its adverse effects can. Improvements in mobility are possible for the more immobile older adults. Relatively small improvements in mobility can decrease the incidence and severity of complications and improve the well being of the elderly. Any physical activity is better than none and should be encouraged. Being involved in meaningful activities often leads to improved self-esteem, self-worth, recognition, friendships, enjoyment, improved physical health, and/or independence, all of which enhance the quality of life and contribute to wellbeing.

Patient's Issues and Objectives	Consultation Assessment and Plan	Signature	Date	Review Date
Mobility and physical activity To promote and encourage mobilisation and participation in physical activity	1. Discuss the importance of physical activity with the patient and, or relative and agree the plan of care.			
	2. Note any concerns or anxieties they have:			
	3. Highlight the **patient's ability to move or assist with moving and transferring:** | ABLE TO WEIGHT BEAR | | PARTIALLY ABLE TO WEIGHT BEAR | CAN WEIGHT BEAR FOR SHORT PERIODS | UNABLE TO WEIGHT BEAR | | IMMOBILE |..			
	4. Note if the patient is in pain or suffers from a painful condition:			
	5. Detail any physical disability or health issues which may restrict the patient moving or participating in physical activity:			
	6. Highlight how the patient mobilises:| WALKS INDEPENDENTLY | WALKS WIH A STICK | WALKS WITH A ZIMMER | | WALKS WITH A ROLLATOR ZIMMER | REQUIRES SUPERVISION | RQUIRES ENCOURAGEMENT | | REQUIRES ASSISTANCE OF ONE | REQUIRES ASSISTANCE OF TWO | REQUIRES FREQUENT REST PERIODS | | IMMOBILE |			
	7. Detail the distance the patient can comfortably walk:			

Copynght © 2020 Planning For Care Limited

CARE PLAN: Mobility and Physical Activity

This care plan must be reviewed monthly (or more often if required) and each action must be signed and dated

Patient's Issues and Objectives	Consultation Assessment and Plan	Signature	Date	Review Date
	8. Note the agreed plan of care **for the patient to mobilise, walk or exercise**:			
	9. Note if the patient has any issues with memory or understanding:			
	10. Liaise with the patient's General Practitioner, physiotherapist or healthcare worker, as necessary.			

Name	Patient/Relative Signature	Date

Copyright © 2020 Planning For Care Limited

CARE PLAN: Motor Neurone Disease

This care plan must be reviewed monthly (or more often if required) and each action must be signed and dated

Motor neurone disease, MND, is a progressive condition that damages the nerves in the brain and spinal cord, leaving muscles wasted and weak. Over time the cells responsible for transmitting the chemical messages, which enable muscle movements, become injured and subsequently die. This causes muscle weakness and wasting to develop. The muscles of the hands, arms and legs are usually affected first. The affected muscles may become twitchy and stiff, and painful cramps may occur from time to time. As the disease progresses, the muscles of the mouth and throat may be affected. Speech may become slurred and swallowing may be difficult, resulting in food particles finding their way into the lungs, causing recurrent chest infections. Neck muscles become weakened. Eventually, the disease interferes with the muscles involved in breathing. Although treatments can be given to make breathing easier, respiratory failure is usually the cause of death in this terminal illness.

Patient's Issues and Objectives	Consultation Assessment and Plan	Signature	Date	Review Date
Motor Neurone Disease To promote effective management of the condition To maintain an optimal level of independence and lifestyle	**1. Discuss the condition with the patient and, or relative and agree the plan of care.**			
	2. Note the patient's and, or relative's understanding of the condition and any concerns they have:			
	3. Highlight any issues or symptoms experienced by the patient: | PAIN | MUSCLE CRAMPS | MUSCLE SPASMS | DIFFICULTY WITH SPEECH | DIFFICULTY SWALLOWING | DEPRESSION | | EXCESS SALIVA | DIFFICULTY BREATHING | EMOTIONAL ISSUES | COGNITIVE ISSUES | DIFFICULTY WITH MOBILITY | | DIFFICULTY WITH DEXTERITY | OTHER:			
	4. Note any issues the patient has with speech or communication and the agreed plan of care to address this:			
	5. Note any issues the patient has with swallowing and the agreed plan of care to address this:			
	6. Note any psychological or emotional issues and the agreed plan of care to address them:			
	7. Note any issues with the patient's mobility and the agreed plan of care to address them:			
	8. Note if the patient suffers from fatigue and the agreed plan of care to address this:			

Copyright © 2020 Planning For Care Limited

CARE PLAN: Motor Neurone Disease

This care plan must be reviewed monthly (or more often if required) and each action must be signed and dated

Patient's Issues and Objectives	Consultation Assessment and Plan	Signature	Date	Review Date
	9. Note any issues with the patient's coordination and the agreed plan of care to address this:			
	10. Highlight any specialised equipment that may assist the patient: | ANTI SPILLAGE CUP | ADAPTED CUTLERY | MECHANICAL HELPING HAND | NON SLIP TABLE MATS | PLATE GUARDS | | PICTURE BOARD | ALPHABET BOARD |...............................			
	11. Note the prescribed medication, dose and frequency to alleviate symptoms:			
	12. Liaise with the General Practitioner as necessary.			

Name	Patient/Relative Signature	Date

Copyright © 2020 Planning For Care Limited

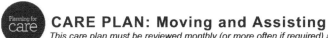

CARE PLAN: Moving and Assisting

This care plan must be reviewed monthly (or more often if required) and each action must be signed and dated

The Manual Handling Operations Regulations 1992, as amended require that a risk assessment must be completed to avoid hazardous manual handling operations when moving or assisting a patient. Other factors have to be considered when preparing to move a patient safely, such as the health and physical condition of the patient, the environment, position of bed and the bed height, and sufficiency of space for the nurse or carer to set the patient into the correct position prior to the lift. It is important for the nurse or carer to re assess the circumstances prior to any lift and if they have any concerns, they should seek advice.

Patient's Issues and Objectives	Consultation Assessment and Plan	Signature	Date	Review Date
Moving and assisting To move or transfer the patient safely and without injury to the patient or the person carrying out the move	1. Discuss with the patient and, or the relative any risks identified in the moving and handling risk assessment.			
	2. Detail the main factors identified in the risk assessment which indicate the need for the patient to be assisted in moving or transferring safely:			
	3. Note the agreed plan for moving or transferring the patient and the equipment which must be used for the safety of the patient and the employee:			
	4. Note if the patient and, or the relative have any concerns or anxieties regarding the equipment or plan of care:			
	5. Note if the patient has any cognitive issues, or any other issues, which may cause a risk to his or her safety when being transferred or moved:			
	6. Note the agreed plan of care to overcome any issues which the patient has as identified above:			

Copyright © 2020 Planning For Care Limited

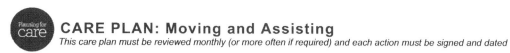

CARE PLAN: Moving and Assisting

This care plan must be reviewed monthly (or more often if required) and each action must be signed and dated

Patient's Issues and Objectives	Consultation Assessment and Plan	Signature	Date	Review Date
	7. Specify the assistance the patient requires for showering or bathing:			

Name	Patient/Relative Signature	Date

CARE PLAN: MRSA (Methicillin Resistant Staphylococcus Aureus) Positive

This care plan must be reviewed monthly (or more often if required) and each action must be signed and dated

MRSA stands for Methicillin Resistant Staphylococcus Aureus, which is a common skin bacteria, that is resistant to a range of antibiotics. The MRSA bacteria live on the skin of one in three people and are often transferred onto other surfaces. About 1 in 100 is a carrier of MRSA, it is not normally a problem for the person carrying the bacteria unless they have a cut, wound or broken skin. However, they are at risk of spreading it to more vulnerable people. MRSA usually poses little risk to healthy people. The elderly, very young or the unwell are most at risk as their immune systems are weakened. MRSA infections are transmitted from person to person by direct contact with the skin clothing or hard surfaces that had recent physical contact with a person infected with MRSA.

Patient's Issues and Objectives	Consultation Assessment and Plan	Signature	Date	Review Date
MRSA Positive To effectively promote recovery and alleviate any concerns To prevent cross infection or contamination	1. Discuss the MRSA infection with the patient and, or relative and agree the plan of care.			
	2. Explain the importance of infection control measures, which will be implemented.			
	3. Note the patient's and, or relative's understanding of the condition and any concerns and anxieties they have:			
	4. Specify the area(s) where MRSA is present:			
	5. Consult with the General Practitioner regarding the positive MRSA swab and note any prescribed treatment:			
	6. Ensure all staff including domestic staff are informed of the infection and wear protective gloves and aprons whilst carrying out personal care, cleaning the room and toilet areas. Environmental cleaning must be increased paying particular attention to toilet areas, bathroom door handles and support rails.			
	7. If MRSA is present in a wound site, the wound must be kept covered with the prescribed dressing.			
	8. 48 hours after the completion of treatment, the affected area should be swabbed again and sent to the laboratory for analysis. Note the result of first swab:			
	9. Then 72 hours after the completion of the treatment another swab should be sent to the laboratory for analysis. Note the result of second swab:			
	10. If MRSA is still present consult the patient's General Practitioner			
	11. Note any further treatment plan:			

Copyright © 2020 Planning For Care Limited

CARE PLAN: MRSA (Methicillin Resistant Staphylococcus Aureus) Positive
This care plan must be reviewed monthly (or more often if required) and each action must be signed and dated

Patient's Issues and Objectives	Consultation Assessment and Plan	Signature	Date	Review Date
	12. Ensure good hand washing techniques are used by all staff, patient and visitors.			
	13. Ensure all clothing is put into alginate bags and sealed before leaving the patient's room.			
	14. Ensure excellent personal hygiene standards are maintained.			
	15. Monitor the patient's condition and liaise with the General Practitioner as required.			

Name	Patient/Relative Signature	Date

CARE PLAN: Multiple Sclerosis

This care plan must be reviewed monthly (or more often if required) and each action must be signed and dated

Multiple sclerosis, MS, is a disease affecting the nerves of the brain and spinal cord. Each nerve fibre in the brain and spinal cord is surrounded by a protective layer of protein called myelin In MS the myelin becomes damaged, consequently, the electrical impulses that travel along the nerves become slower. In addition, the nerves themselves are damaged. This can cause a wide range of potential symptoms, such as loss of vision, or blurring vision, spasticity, muscle weakness and tightness, pain, difficulties with movement, balance and co-ordination, fatigue, numbness and tingling. Treatment for MS can be split into three main categories treatment for relapses of MS symptoms, steroids, treatment for specific MS symptoms and treatment to slow the progression of MS, disease-modifying medicines.

Patient's Issues and Objectives	Consultation Assessment and Plan	Signature	Date	Review Date
Multiple Sclerosis To promote effective management of the condition To maintain an optimal level of independence and lifestyle	1. Discuss the condition with the patient and, or relative and agree the plan of care.			
	2. Note the patient's and, or the relative's understanding of the condition and any concerns or anxieties they have:			
	3. Note the patient's past history of Multiple Sclerosis if available:			
	4. Highlight the symptoms the patient experiences: | FATIGUE | DIFFICULTY WALKING | LOSS OF VISION | | BLURRED VISION | PROBLEMS CONTROLLING THE BLADDER | NUMBNESS AND TINGLING | MUSCLE STIFFNESS | | MUSCLE SPASMS | MUSCLE WEAKNESS | DIFFICULTIES WITH BALANCE AND CO-ORDINATION | BOWEL ISSUES | | PROBLEMS WITH THINKING, LEARNING AND PLANNING | PAIN | DEPRESSION | ANXIETY | SEXUAL PROBLEMS | | SPEECH DIFFICULTIES | SWALLOWING DIFFICULTIES |			
	5. Note any issues such as anxiety or depression and the agreed plan of care to address them:			
	6. Note if the patient has pain and specify the location, type and frequency:			
	7. Note any issues the patient has with vision and the agreed plan of care to address them:			
	8. Note any issues the patient has with mobility and the agreed plan of care to address this:			
	9. Note any issues with the patient's coordination or dexterity and the agreed plan of care to address this:			

Copyright © 2020 Planning For Care Limited

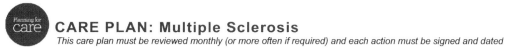

CARE PLAN: Multiple Sclerosis

This care plan must be reviewed monthly (or more often if required) and each action must be signed and dated

Patient's Issues and Objectives	Consultation Assessment and Plan	Signature	Date	Review Date
	10. Highlight any specialised equipment that may assist the patient:	ANTI SPILLAGE CUP	ADAPTED CUTLERY		MECHANICAL HELPING HAND	NON-SLIP TABLE MATS	PLATE GUARDS	WALKING AID	………………………………..			
	11. Note any bladder issues and the agreed plan of care to address this:			
	12. Note any bowel issues and the agreed plan of care to address this:			
	13. Note if the patient has any other issues due to the condition and the agreed plan of care to address them:			
	14. Note the prescribed medication, dose and frequency:			
	15. Liaise with the General Practitioner as necessary.			

Name	Patient/Relative Signature	Date

Copyright © 2020 Planning For Care Limited

CARE PLAN: Muscle Cramps
This care plan must be reviewed monthly (or more often if required) and each action must be signed and dated

Muscle cramps are sudden, involuntary contractions, which can occur in muscles. An intense, sudden, sharp pain, lasting from a few seconds to fifteen minutes, is the most common symptom. The most commonly affected muscles are in the lower leg and, the thigh, but it can also affect the abdominal wall, arms, hands, and feet. It can result from overuse of muscles while exercising, or from muscle injuries, dehydration or low levels of calcium and potassium. Poor blood supply to the legs and feet can cause cramping in those areas when exercising, walking, or participating in physical activities. Some conditions, which can result in muscle cramps, include spinal nerve compression, alcoholism, pregnancy, kidney failure, and low thyroid gland function. Muscle cramps are usually harmless, however, medical advice should be sought if they are severe, interrupt sleep, do not improve with stretching, or persist for long periods as this could be due to an underlying medical condition.

Patient's Issues and Objectives	Consultation Assessment and Plan	Signature	Date	Review Date
Muscle Cramps To minimise the occurrence of muscle cramps and where possible treat the underlying cause	**1.** Discuss the muscle cramps with the patient and, or relatives and agree plan of care.			
	2. Note the patient's and, or relatives understanding of the condition and any concerns or anxieties they have:			
	3. Note the past history of muscle cramps, when they first started, how frequently they occur and any treatment received:			
	4. Highlight the cause of the patient's muscle cramps if known: | EXERCISE | MUSCLE INJURY | NEUROLOGICAL CONDITION | MOTOR NEURONE DISEASE | LIVER DISEASE | TOXINS | | PERIPHERAL NEUROPATHY | INFECTION | DEHYDRATION | DIURETICS | RALOXIFENE | NICOTINIC ACID | NIFEDIPINE | | STATINS |..			
	5. Note the area(s) of the body the patient experiences muscle cramps, when they occur, how frequently, and how long they last:			
	6. Note if the patient's sleep is interrupted or disturbed as a result of muscle cramps:			
	7. Consult with the General Practitioner for advice and detail the advice:			

Copyright © 2020 Planning For Care Limited

CARE PLAN: Muscle Cramps

This care plan must be reviewed monthly (or more often if required) and each action must be signed and dated

Patient's Issues and Objectives	Consultation Assessment and Plan	Signature	Date	Review Date
	8. Note the prescribed medication, dose and frequency:			
	9. Encourage adequate fluid intake 1500-2000 mls per day.			
	10. Note if the patient has any issues drinking adequate fluids, detail any assistance required, and the agreed plan of care:			
	11. Liaise with the General Practitioner as required.			

Name	Patient/Relative Signature	Date

Copyright © 2020 Planning For Care Limited

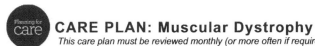

CARE PLAN: Muscular Dystrophy

This care plan must be reviewed monthly (or more often if required) and each action must be signed and dated

Muscular dystrophies, MD, are a group of inherited genetic conditions, which gradually cause the muscles to weaken, leading to an increased level of disablement. It often begins by affecting a particular group of muscles before affecting the muscles more widely. Some types eventually affect the heart or the muscles used for breathing, at which point the condition becomes life threatening. There is currently no cure for MD, but treatment can help manage many of the symptoms. Duchenne muscular dystrophy usually affects boys in early childhood, and men with this condition only live to 20 or 30. Myotonic dystrophy can result in a mask-like expressionless face, premature balding, cataracts, and heart irregularities and can develop at any age. Facioscapulohumeral muscular dystrophy results in slowly progressive weakness of the muscles of the face, shoulders, and feet. Becker muscular dystrophy develops later in childhood. Limb-girdle muscular dystrophy results in a progressive weakness and wasting of the muscles in the hips or shoulders. Oculopharyngeal muscular dystrophy begins in the muscles of the eyes and throat, usually appearing around the age 40 to 60, and it progresses slowly. Emery-Dreifuss muscular dystrophy, progresses slowly and begins in the upper arms or upper legs. Contractures of the limbs are common, as are serious heart problems.

Patient's Issues and Objectives	Consultation Assessment and Plan	Signature	Date	Review Date
Muscular Dystrophy To promote effective management of the condition To maintain an optimal level of independence and lifestyle	1. Discuss the condition with the patient and, or relative and agree the plan of care.			
	2. Note the patient's and, or relative's understanding of the condition and any concerns they have:			
	3. Note the past medical history of muscular dystrophy, the type, when it was diagnosed and treatment received:			
	4. Highlight any issues or symptoms experienced by the patient: | MUSCLE WEAKNESS | MUSCLE WASTING | MUSCLE STIFFNESS | MUSCLE ACHES | MUSCLE CRAMPS | CATARACTS | | UNSTEADY GAIT | EXCESSIVE FATIGUE | CONTRACTURE OF JOINTS | DIFFICULTY SWALLOWING | DROOPY EYELIDS | | DEPRESSION | DIFFICULTY SPEAKING | DIFFICULTY BREATHING | IRREGULAR HEARTBEAT | PSYCHOLOGICAL |			
	5. Note the affected areas of muscle weakness:			
	6. Note the agreed plan of care for muscle exercise and mobility, as advised by the physiotherapist and any issues:			
	7. Note any issues the patient has with breathing and the agreed plan to address this:			

Copyright © 2020 Planning For Care Limited

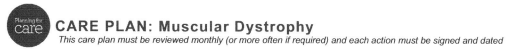

CARE PLAN: Muscular Dystrophy

This care plan must be reviewed monthly (or more often if required) and each action must be signed and dated

Patient's Issues and Objectives	Consultation Assessment and Plan	Signature	Date	Review Date
	8. Note any issues the patient has with speaking or swallowing and the agreed plan of care to address this:			
	9. Note if the patient suffers from fatigue and the agreed plan of care to address this:			
	10. Note any issues with the patient's vision and the agreed plan of care to address this:			
	11. Note if the patient has muscle pain and, or cramps and specify the location and frequency:			
	12. Note any emotional or psychological issues and the agreed plan to address them:			
	13. Note the prescribed medication, dose and frequency:			
	14. Monitor the patient's condition and liaise with the General Practitioner as necessary.			

Name	Patient/Relative Signature	Date

Copyright © 2020 Planning For Care Limited

CARE PLAN: Myasthenia Gravis

This care plan must be reviewed monthly (or more often if required) and each action must be signed and dated

Myasthenia gravis literally means 'grave muscle weakness'. It can affect muscles that control eye and eyelid movement, facial expression, chewing, swallowing and talking, the muscles in the arms, fingers, neck and legs and can cause unstable gait. Less often, the muscles involved in breathing may be affected. Muscles of the heart and other vital organs are not affected. The immune system produces antibodies which block or damage muscle receptors resulting in poor transmission of nerve impulses to the muscles, which do not contract well and become weak. The weakness can be made worse by physical activity and improved by rest. It can be exacerbated with stress, hot water, fever, overexertion and infection. A myasthenia crisis occurs when the muscles controlling breathing weaken to the point that ventilation is inadequate, creating a medical emergency. When the muscles used for speaking, chewing and swallowing are affected it may be beneficial to eat softer foods and avoid foods which require to be chewed, to eat when the muscles are at their strongest and to eat smaller meals more often, resting between mouthfuls. It may be beneficial to plan activities to coincide with a time energy levels at their highest. This may be early in the day or after taking medication.

Patient's Issues and Objectives	Consultation Assessment and Plan	Signature	Date	Review Date
Myasthenia Gravis To promote effective management of the condition To maintain an optimal level of independence and lifestyle	1. Discuss the condition with the patient and, or relative and agree the plan of care.			
	2. Note the patient's and, or relative's understanding of the condition and any concerns or anxieties they have:			
	3. Note the past medical history of Myasthenia gravis, when it was diagnosed and the treatment received:			
	4. Note the affected areas of muscle weakness:			
	5. Note any issues the patient has with vision and the agreed plan of care to address this:			
	6. Note any issues the patient has with communication and the agreed plan of care to address this:			

CARE PLAN: Myasthenia Gravis

This care plan must be reviewed monthly (or more often if required) and each action must be signed and dated

Patient's Issues and Objectives	Consultation Assessment and Plan	Signature	Date	Review Date
	7. Note any issues the patient has with nutrition and the agreed plan of care to address this:			
	8. Note any issues the patient has with mobility and the agreed plan of care to address this:			
	9. Note any other issues expressed by the patient due to his, or her condition:			
	10. Note the patient's prescribed medication, dose and frequency:			
	11. Monitor the patient's condition and consult with the General Practitioner if required.			

Name	Patient/Relative Signature	Date

Copyright © 2020 Planning For Care Limited

CARE PLAN: Nutritional Intake

This care plan must be reviewed monthly (or more often if required) and each action must be signed and dated

Food provides energy and nutrients that the body needs to stay healthy. Nutrients include proteins, carbohydrates, fats, vitamins and water. The benefits of healthy eating include mental awareness, resistance to illness and disease, higher energy levels, a more robust immune system, faster recuperation times and better management of chronic illness.

Patient's Issues and Objectives	Consultation Assessment and Plan	Signature	Date	Review Date
Nutritional Intake **To promote a healthy nutritional intake**	1. Discuss nutritional requirements with the patient and, or relative and agree the plan of care.			
	2. Note any preferences, portion sizes or specific issues with the patient's dietary intake and the agreed plan of care:			
	3. Highlight the preferred or recommended consistency of food: | NORMAL | SOFT | PUREED | THICKENED FLUIDS |			
	4. Highlight the assistance the patient requires for eating: | INDEPENDENT | NEEDS ENCOURAGEMENT | | NEEDS FOOD CUT UP | NEEDS ASSISTANCE | VARIES DAILY | ASSESS NEEDS DAILY |.............................			
	5. Highlight what assistance the patient needs choosing food: | INDEPENDENT | NEEDS ENCOURAGEMENT | | NEEDS HELP | VARIES DAILY | CONSULT RELATIVE TO CHOOSE PATIENT'S PREFERENCES FROM MENU |			
	6. Highlight breakfast preference: | CEREAL | PORRIDGE | SUGAR | HONEY | JAM | MARMALADE | TOAST | | BOILED EGGS | FRIED EGGS| SCRAMBLED EGGS | BACON | SAUSAGE | BREAD ROLL |.............................			
	7. Highlight lunch preference: | SOUP | BREAD | MEAT | POULTRY | FISH | PASTA | BOILED POTATOES | CHIPS | | MASHED POTATOES | ROAST POTATOES | RICE | VEGETABLES |.............................			
	8. Highlight dinner preference: | SOUP | MEAT | POULTRY | FISH | VEGETABLES | RICE | PASTA | BOILED POTATOES | | MASHED POTATOES | ROAST POTATO | CHIPS | EGGS | SANDWICHES | YOGHURT | CAKES | SMOOTHIES | FRUIT |			
	9. Note the patient's favourite foods and snacks to eat:			
	10. Complete a nutritional assessment and review monthly.			
	11. Record the patient's weight: Body Mass Index (BMI):			

Copyright © 2020 Planning For Care Limited

CARE PLAN: Nutritional Intake

This care plan must be reviewed monthly (or more often if required) and each action must be signed and dated

Patient's Issues and Objectives	Consultation Assessment and Plan	Signature	Date	Review Date
	12. Malnutrition Universal Screening Tool, MUST Score:			
	13. Note any specialised aids required for eating and any issues the patient has:			
	14. Highlight the frequency of monitoring the patient's weight: | MONTHLY | WEEKLY | AS NECESSARY |			
	15. Ensure all food is attractive and well presented and is of appropriate consistency.			
	16. Note who the patient prefers to dine with, and where:			

Name	Patient/Relative Signature	Date

Copyright © 2020 Planning For Care Limited

CARE PLAN: Nutritional Intake Inadequate

This care plan must be reviewed monthly (or more often if required) and each action must be signed and dated

Food provides energy and nutrients that the body needs to stay healthy. Nutrients include proteins, carbohydrates, fats, vitamins and water. The benefits of healthy eating include mental awareness, resistance to illness and disease, higher energy levels, a more robust immune system, faster recuperation times and better management of chronic illness.

Patient's Issues and Objectives	Consultation Assessment and Plan	Signature	Date	Review Date
Nutritional Intake is inadequate **To maximise nutritional intake and maintain a healthy diet**	1. Discuss the issue with the patient and, or relative and agree the plan of care.			
	2. Note the patient's and, or relative's understanding of the issue and any concerns or anxieties they have:			
	3. Note any previous history of poor dietary intake:			
	4. Note any preferences, portion sizes or specific issues with the patient's dietary intake and the agreed plan of care:			
	5. Highlight the preferred or recommended consistency of food:	NORMAL	SOFT	PUREED	THICKENED FLUIDS				
	6. Highlight the assistance the patient requires for eating:	INDEPENDENT	NEEDS ENCOURAGEMENT TO EAT		NEEDS FOOD CUT UP	NEEDS ASSISTANCE	ASSISTANCE VARIES FROM DAY TO DAY	ASSESS NEEDS DAILY				
	7. Highlight what assistance the patient needs choosing food:	INDEPENDENT	NEEDS ENCOURAGEMENT		NEEDS HELP	VARIES DAILY	CONSULT RELATIVE TO CHOOSE PATIENT'S PREFERENCES FROM MENU				
	8. Highlight breakfast preference:	CEREAL	PORRIDGE	SUGAR	HONEY	JAM	MARMALADE	TOAST	SAUSAGE		BACON	BOILED EGGS	FRIED EGGS	SCRAMBLED EGGS	BREAD ROLL	....			
	9. Highlight lunch preference:	SOUP	BREAD	MEAT	POULTRY	FISH	PASTA	RICE	BOILED POTATOES	CHIPS		MASHED POTATOES	ROAST POTATOES	VEGETABLES	....			
	10. Highlight dinner preference:	SOUP	MEAT	POULTRY	FISH	RICE	PASTA	VEGETABLES	ROAST POTATOES		BOILED POTATOES	MASHED POTATOES	CHIPS	EGGS	SANDWICHES	YOGHURT	CAKES	SMOOTHIES	FRUIT	....			
	11. Note the patient's favourite foods and snacks to eat, if reluctant for normal diet:			

Copyright © 2020 Planning For Care Limited

CARE PLAN: Nutritional Intake Inadequate

This care plan must be reviewed monthly (or more often if required) and each action must be signed and dated

Patient's Issues and Objectives	Consultation Assessment and Plan	Signature	Date	Review Date
	12. Complete a nutritional assessment and review monthly.			
	13. Record the patient's weight Body Mass Index (BMI):			
	14. Malnutrition Universal Screening Tool (MUST Score):			
	15. Specify the agreed plan for improving dietary intake, such as a fortified diet, adding cheese, cream, sugar or honey:			
	16. Note any specialised aids required for eating and any issues:			
	17. Note any prescribed supplements and the frequency:			
	18. Highlight the frequency of monitoring the patient's weight: | MONTHLY | WEEKLY | AS NECESSARY |			
	19. Ensure all food is attractive and well presented and is of appropriate consistency.			
	20. Note where the patient prefers to dine and with which friends:			
	21. If necessary commence on fluid and diet chart and liaise with the General Practitioner and the Dietician.			

Name	Patient/Relative Signature	Date

Copyright © 2020 Planning For Care Limited

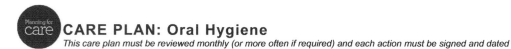

CARE PLAN: Oral Hygiene

This care plan must be reviewed monthly (or more often if required) and each action must be signed and dated

Oral Hygiene is the practice of keeping the mouth and teeth clean to prevent dental problems especially dental caries, gingivitis and bad breath. Thrush presents as white patches in the mouth tongue or cheeks when they are brushed away it reveals a reddened tender area that may bleed slightly. Mouth ulcers are painful sores inside the mouth that can appear on the tongue or gums or inside the cheek and lips. The ulcer, which is usually circular with a yellow or white centre and a raised red rim, is an area where the surface of the mouth's lining has been removed. This means that nerve cells are exposed causing pain and discomfort particularly when eating certain foods.

Patient's Issues and Objectives	Consultation Assessment and Plan	Signature	Date	Review Date
Oral Hygiene To maintain a high standard of oral hygiene	1. Discuss the issue with the patient and, or relative and agree the plan of care.			
	2. Note the patient's and, or relative's understanding of the issue and any concerns or anxieties they have:			
	3. Note if the patient has their own teeth or dentures and any previous history of oral hygiene issues:			
	4. Note the patient's preferred toothpaste:			
	5. Note the patient's preferred toothbrush:			
	6. Highlight the reason for the care plan: • dehydration and dryness of the mucosa, the lining of the mouth, due to inadequate fluid intake • poor cellular repair and vitamin deficiencies, due to poor nutritional intake • insufficient saliva production, leading to infection and dryness to the lining of the mouth • dementia or lack of motivation in maintaining oral hygiene OTHER:			
	7. Note the plan to alleviate or improve the contributing factors:			
	8. Highlight if there is evidence of changes in the mouth: | BLEEDING | ULCERS | PAIN INFECTION | THRUSH | | LACK OF SALIVA |			
	9. Note any prescribed medication, dose and frequency:			

Copyright © 2020 Planning For Care Limited

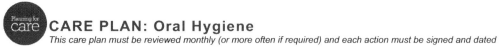

CARE PLAN: Oral Hygiene

This care plan must be reviewed monthly (or more often if required) and each action must be signed and dated

Patient's Issues and Objectives	Consultation Assessment and Plan	Signature	Date	Review Date
	10. Highlight the level of assistance the patient requires with oral hygiene: <ul><li>encourage the patient to brush teeth, own, or dentures, to rinse mouth after meals and last thing before retiring</li><li>assist the patient to brush teeth, own or dentures, to rinse mouth after meals and last thing before retiring</li><li>soak dentures overnight in water or a mild denture-soaking solution they must remain moist to keep their shape</li><li>maximum assistance with cleaning teeth and the lining of the mouth and tongue</li></ul> SPECIFY: …………………………………………………………………………………			
	11. Where maximum assistance is required highlight the equipment to be used: | ORAL HYGIENE TRAY | MOUTH SWABS TO BE KEPT IN PATIENT'S ROOM | MOUTH WASH AS PRESCRIBED | | BICARBONATE OF SODA | GLOVES | OTHER: ………………………………………			
	12. Note the frequency of mouth care: ………………………………………………………………………………………………………			
	13. Ensure the oral hygiene tray is removed and changed each day.			
	14. Ensure the patient's own toothbrush is replaced 3 monthly and that they have toothpaste of their choice.			
	15. Monitor effectiveness of oral hygiene and liaise with the dentist and General Practitioner as required. ……………………………………………………………………………………………………… ……………………………………………………………………………………………………… ……………………………………………………………………………………………………… ……………………………………………………………………………………………………… ……………………………………………………………………………………………………… ………………………………………………………………………………………………………			

Name	Patient /Relative Signature	Date

Copyright © 2020 Planning For Care Limited

CARE PLAN: Oral Thrush

This care plan must be reviewed monthly (or more often if required) and each action must be signed and dated

Oral thrush is a yeast infection in the mouth, caused by a type of fungus called Candida albicans. It causes an unpleasant taste, soreness, a burning sensation on the tongue and difficulty swallowing. Oral thrush is not contagious, meaning it cannot be passed to others. Candida albicans fungus is naturally found in the mouth in small amounts. Oral thrush develops when these levels increase. This can be the result of a taking certain medications, particularly inhaled steroids, poor oral hygiene, smoking, or a weakened immune system, for example due to HIV or AIDS. Around 7 in 10 people who wear dentures will get oral thrush at some stage. Diabetics are also more at risk of developing thrush. Symptoms of oral thrush can include sore, white patches, plaques, in the mouth that can be wiped off, a painful burning sensation on the tongue, a bitter or salty taste in the mouth, redness and soreness on the inside of the mouth and throat, cracks at the corners of the mouth, difficulty swallowing

Patient's Issues And Objectives	Consultation Assessment and Plan	Signature	Date	Review Date
Oral Thrush Promotion and maintenance of a healthy mouth and good oral and dental hygiene	1. Discuss the condition with the patient and, or relative and agree the plan of care.			
	2. Note the patient's and, or relative's understanding of the condition and any concerns or anxieties they have:			
	3. Note any past history of oral thrush and the treatment prescribed:			
	4. Highlight and discuss with the patient and/or the relatives any possible contributing factors: | POOR DENTAL HYGIENE | ILL FITTING DENTURES | POOR ORAL HYGIENE | INFECTION | DIABETES | CANCER | | RADIOTHERAPY | CHEMOTHERAPY | ANTIBIOTIC THERAPY | MEDICATION, INHALED STERIODS | SMOKING | | IRON DEFICIENCY ANAEMIA | PERNICIOUS ANAEMIA |			
	5. Note the agreed plan of care to address any of the contributing factors:			
	6. Highlight the symptoms experienced by the patient: | SORE WHITE OR YELLOW PATCHES IN THE MOUTH THAT CAN BE SCRAPED OFF | PATCHES ON THE TONGUE | | PATCHES INSIDE OF THE CHEEKS | BURNING SENSATION ON THE TONGUE | DIFFICULTY SWALLOWING | | BITTER OR SALTY TASTE | REDNESS OR SORENESS MOUTH AND THROAT | CRACKS AT CORNERS OF MOUTH |			
	7. Consult with the patient's General Practitioner.			

Copyright © 2020 Planning For Care Limited

CARE PLAN: Oral Thrush

This care plan must be reviewed monthly (or more often if required) and each action must be signed and dated

Patient's Issues And Objectives	Consultation Assessment and Plan	Signature	Date	Review Date
	8. Note the prescribed medication, dosage, and treatment regime:			
	9. Monitor the effectiveness of the treatment and the condition of the patient's mouth.			
	10. Highlight the agreed plan of care for good oral hygiene: | HEALTHY DIET | RINSE MOUTH AFTER MEALS | REGULAR DENTAL CHECKS | BRUSHING TEETH AFTER MEALS | | CLEANING DENTURES AFTER MEALS | REGULAR FLOSSING | USING MOUTHWASH REGULARLY | SPECIFY:			
	10. Liaise with the patient's General Practitioner as required.			

Name	Patient/Relative Signature	Date

CARE PLAN: Osteoarthritis

This care plan must be reviewed monthly (or more often if required) and each action must be signed and dated

Osteoarthritis is sometimes called 'wear and tear' arthritis and becomes more likely as a person gets older. Being overweight increases the risk of osteoarthritis, particularly of the knee. An injury, operation, earlier disease or repeated strain at a joint may lead to osteoarthritis later in life. The smooth cartilage that takes the strain in a normal joint becomes rough, brittle and weak and to compensate, the bone beneath thickens and spreads out, forming knobbly outgrowths. The membrane surrounding the joint thickens and the fluid-filled space within it becomes smaller often resulting in inflammation. As osteoarthritis gets worse, bits of cartilage may break away from the one, causing the bone ends to rub together and the ligaments to become strained. This causes a lot of pain and changes the shape of the joint. It is most common in the hands, knees, hips and feet, but can develop in the back and neck. The condition causes joints to become stiff and painful to move, It usually develops slowly and the changes can be so gradual. The condition usually settles down after a number of years and, although the joints may have a knobbly appearance, they may become less painful.

Patient's Issues and Objectives	Consultation Assessment and Plan	Signature	Date	Review Date
Osteoarthritis To minimise pain and discomfort to promote effective management of the condition To maintain an optimal level of independence and lifestyle	1. Discuss the condition with the patient and, or relative and agree the plan of care.			
	2. Note the patient's and, or relative's understanding of the condition and any concerns or anxieties they have:			
	3. Note the past medical history of osteoarthritis, when it was diagnosed and the prescribed treatment:			
	4. Note the areas affected:			
	5. Highlight any signs and symptoms experienced by the patient: • joint tenderness • increased pain and stiffness when joints have not moved for a while • joints appearing slightly larger or more 'knobbly' than usual • a grating or crackling sound or sensation in the joints • limited range of movement in the joints • weakness and muscle wasting, loss of muscle bulk			
	6. Highlight any issues the patient has with the activities of daily living, as a result of osteoarthritis: | MOBILITY | GETTING UP IN THE MORNING | GOING TO BED SLEEPING DUE TO PAIN | EATING AND DRINKING | | INCONTINENCE DUE TO REDUCED MOBILITY | CONSTIPATION DUE TO ANALGESIA | DRESSING | ACTIVITIES | OTHER:...			

Copyright © 2020 Planning For Care Limited

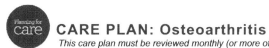

CARE PLAN: Osteoarthritis

This care plan must be reviewed monthly (or more often if required) and each action must be signed and dated

Patient's Issues and Objectives	Consultation Assessment and Plan	Signature	Date	Review Date
	7. Note the agreed plan of care to assist the patient with any activities of daily living they have issues with:			
	8. Note the prescribed medication, dose and frequency:			
	9. Monitor the condition and liaise with the patient's General Practitioner as required.			

Name	Patient /Relative Signature	Date

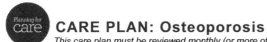

CARE PLAN: Osteoporosis

This care plan must be reviewed monthly (or more often if required) and each action must be signed and date

Osteoporosis is a condition where bones lose density causing them to become weak, brittle and more likely to break or fracture. Bones are a living tissue, just like the rest of the body. They consist of cells, which both build and break down bone, within a surrounding substance known as the extracellular matrix, which is composed of proteins and mineralised components. The composition of the extracellular matrix determines how strong the bone is, and the higher the concentration of calcium, the greater the strength. Bone reaches a peak of being most dense and strong by around the third decade of life. From this point, bone mass slowly decreases.

Patient's Issues and Objectives	Consultation Assessment and Plan	Signature	Date	Review Date
Osteoporosis To manage osteoporosis and minimise risk of fracture.	1. Discuss the condition with the patient and, or relative and agree the plan of care.			
	2. Note the patient's and, or relative's understanding of the condition and any concerns or anxieties they have:			
	3. Ensure a high risk of falls care plan is completed and in place for the patient.			
	4. Encourage the patient to take fluids and a diet rich in calcium, vitamin D and protein.			
	5. Encourage the patient to exercise regularly each day. Note if the patient has issues with mobility and specify any assistance required:			
	6. Note the prescribed medication, dose and frequency of administration:			
	7. Alendronic Acid and Risedronate must be taken 30 minutes before food or drink in the morning.			
	8. Review the patient's falls risk assessment monthly and modify the care plan accordingly.			
	9. Liaise with the patient's General Practitioner where appropriate.			
	....			

Copyright © 2020 Planning For Care Limited

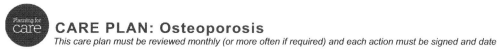

CARE PLAN: Osteoporosis

This care plan must be reviewed monthly (or more often if required) and each action must be signed and date

Patient's Issues and Objectives	Consultation Assessment and Plan	Signature	Date	Review Date

Name	Patient/Relative Signature	Date

Copyright © 2020 Planning For Care Limited

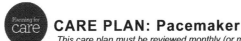

CARE PLAN: Pacemaker

This care plan must be reviewed monthly (or more often if required) and each action must be signed and dated

A pacemaker is a small device, which is surgically placed in the chest or abdomen to help control abnormal heart rhythms. It uses low-energy electrical pulses to prompt the heart to beat at a normal rate. They are used to treat irregular rhythm where the heart can beat too fast, tachycardia, or too slow, bradycardia. Most pacemakers have a special sensor that recognises body movement or breathing rate, allowing them to speed up the discharge rate when active. They can relieve some irregular heart beat symptoms, such as tiredness and fainting and can also help a person resume a more active lifestyle. Signs that the pacemaker is not working as it should, or that there may be an infection or blood clot, can include breathlessness, dizziness, fainting, prolonged weakness, swollen arm on the side of the pacemaker, chest pains, prolonged hiccups, a high temperature of 38°C or above, pain, swelling and redness at the site of the pacemaker. The pacemaker is checked regularly to ensure it is working properly and the batteries last between 5 and 15 years and will require to be replaced. It is important that doctors, dentists, and medical technicians are informed of the patient's pacemaker as certain medical procedures can disrupt the pacemaker such as MRI scan, electro cauterisation to stop bleeding during surgery and shockwave lithotripsy for kidney stones. In the event of death it is important to inform the undertakers as the pacemaker can cause an explosion if the patient's body is cremated.

Patient's Issues and Objectives	Consultation Assessment and Plan	Signature	Date	Review Date
Pacemaker To monitor the effects of the pacemaker To maintain an optimal level of health	1. Discuss the pacemaker with the patient and, or relative and agree the plan of care.			
	2. Note the patient's and, or relative's understanding of the pacemaker and any concerns or anxieties they have:			
	3. Discuss the importance of avoiding close or prolonged contact with electrical devices or devices with a strong magnetic fields as these can disrupt the electrical signalling of the pacemaker and prevent it working properly. • Cell phones and MP3 players, for example, iPods • Household appliances, such as microwave ovens • High-tension wires • Metal detectors • Electrical generators			
	4. Discuss the importance of informing all doctors, dentists, and medical technicians of the pacemaker as certain medical procedures can disrupt the pacemaker such as MRI scan, electro cauterisation to stop bleeding during surgery and shockwave lithotripsy for kidney stones.			
	5. Highlight the reason for the pacemaker: | FAST HEARTBEAT | SLOW HEARTBEAT | PREVIOUS HEART ATTACK | ATRIAL FIBRILLATION | HEART FAILURE | | IRREGULAR HEARTBEAT | HEART BLOCK | OTHER...............			
	6. Note the patient's past history of cardiac disease, symptoms experienced, and any treatment received:			
	7. Note the patient's baseline pulse:			

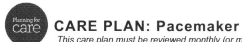

CARE PLAN: Pacemaker

This care plan must be reviewed monthly (or more often if required) and each action must be signed and dated

Patient's Issues and Objectives	Consultation Assessment and Plan	Signature	Date	Review Date
	8. Note when the pacemaker was fitted:			
	9. Note how frequently the clinic requires to check the pacemaker:			
	10. Contact the General Practitioner immediately if there are any signs that the pacemaker is not functioning properly.			

Name	Patient/Relative Signature	Date

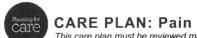

CARE PLAN: Pain

This care plan must be reviewed monthly (or more often if required) and each action must be signed and dated

Pain is an unpleasant sensation that can range from mild discomfort to agony. Pain has both physical and emotional components. The physical part of pain results from nerve stimulation. Pain may be contained to a discrete area, as in an injury, or it can be more diffuse. It is carried by specific nerve fibres, which transmit the pain impulses to the brain. Chronic pain can be extremely emotionally challenging, causing irritation, stress, lack of sleep, and can result in depression. Physical and emotional pain is a major symptom in many medical conditions and can significantly interfere with a person's quality of life, general functioning and ability to recover.

Patient's Issues and Objectives	Consultation Assessment and Plan	Signature	Date	Review Date
Pain To alleviate pain, promote comfort and alleviate associated issues	1. Discuss the issue with the patient and, or relative and agree the plan of care.			
	2. Note any previous medical history and episodes of pain and the treatment prescribed:			
	3. Establish and note if the pain is chronic, indicating how long the patient has had it, or acute and, the type of pain:			
	4. If the patient has dementia and, or is unable to communicate, using observation assess and score the level of pain: a) Vocalisation: whimpering, groaning, crying **0 absent, 1 mild, 2 moderate, 3 severe** b) Facial expression: looking tense, frowning, grimacing, looking frightened **0 absent, 1 mild, 2 moderate, 3 severe** c) Change in body language: fidgeting, rocking, guarding part of the body, withdrawn **0 absent, 1 mild, 2 moderate, 3 severe** d) Behavioural change: increased confusion, refusing to eat, alteration in usual pattern **0 absent, 1 mild, 2 moderate, 3 severe** e) Physiological change: temperature, pulse, high or low blood pressure, perspiring, flushing, pallor **0 absent, 1 mild, 2 moderate, 3 severe** f) Physical changes: skin tears, pressure areas, arthritis, contractures, previous injury **0 absent 1 mild, 2 moderate, 3 severe** **Note the total of the scores for section a-f:** ……………… **(0-2 No Pain, 3-7 Mild Pain, 8-13 Moderate Pain, 14+ Severe Pain)**			
	5. Highlight the severity of pain experienced by the resident: | MILD | INTERMITTENT | MODERATE | SEVERE | VARIES |			
	6. Note the precise location of pain, if it radiates, and where it radiates to:			
	7. Consult with the resident's General Practitioner and note the prescribed medication, dose and frequency:			

Copyright © 2020 Planning For Care Limited

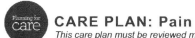

CARE PLAN: Pain

This care plan must be reviewed monthly (or more often if required) and each action must be signed and dated

Patient's Issues and Objectives	Consultation Assessment and Plan	Signature	Date	Review Date
	8. Highlight the agreed plan of care: | ANALGESIA IS GIVEN ROUTINELY AS PRESCRIBED | ANALGESIA IS PRESCRIBED AS REQUIRED |			
	9. If the patient is unable to communicate that they were in pain, specify how they would demonstrate this and when, and in what circumstances, as required pain analgesia should be administered:			
	10. Highlight additional issues experienced due to the pain and ensure a care plan is prepared to address them: | SLEEPLESSNESS | WITHDRAWAL FROM ACTIVITY | INCREASED NEED TO REST | FATIGUE | CHANGES IN MOOD | | DEPRESSION | ANXIETY | STRESS | DISABILITY | LOSS OF APPETITE |			
	11. Encourage the patient to say when they have pain and ask for feedback on the effectiveness of the analgesia.			
	12. Monitor effectiveness of treatment and where necessary liaise with the resident's General Practitioner.			

Name	Resident/Relative Signature	Date

Copyright © 2020 Planning For Care Limited

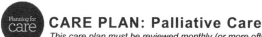

CARE PLAN: Palliative Care

This care plan must be reviewed monthly (or more often if required) and each action must be signed and dated

Palliative care is the active holistic care of patients with advanced progressive illness. Palliative care treats people suffering from serious and chronic illnesses such as cancer, cardiac disease such as congestive heart failure, chronic obstructive pulmonary disease, kidney failure, Alzheimer's, Parkinson's and many more. Management of pain and other symptoms and provision of psychological, social and spiritual support is paramount. The goal of palliative care is achievement of the best quality of life for patients and their families. The aims of palliative care are to affirm life, to integrate psychological and spiritual aspects into mainstream patient care and to provide support to enable patients to live as actively as possible.

Patient's Issues and Objectives	Consultation Assessment and Plan	Signature	Date	Review Date
Palliative Care To assess anticipate and alleviate any symptoms and suffering. To achieve the best quality of life for the patient and their families.	1. Discuss with the patient and, or relative any current physical and emotional issues and agree the plan of care.			
	2. Note the patient's and, or relative's understanding of the issues and any concerns they have:			
	3. Record the patient's past medical history:			
	4. Ensure a palliative care assessment has been completed.			
	5. Highlight any issues experienced by the patient:| PAIN | AGITATION | POOR FLUID INTAKE | BLADDER FUNCTION | | POOR DIETARY INTAKE | NAUSEA | BOWEL FUNCTION | ORAL HYGIENE | RESPIRATORY TRACT SECRETIONS | | BREATHING DIFFICULTIES | PRESSURE AREAS | PRESSURE SORES | DIFFICULTY COMMUNICATING | ISOLATION | | EMOTIONAL ISSUES | FEAR |			
	6. Note any issues with the patient's pain management, and the agreed plan of care to address this:			
	7. Note any issues with the patient's breathing and the agreed plan of care to address this:			
	8. Note any issues with the patients psychological or emotional state and the agreed plan of care to address this:			
	9. Note any issues with the patient's pressure areas and the agreed plan to address this:			

Copyright © 2020 Planning For Care Limited

CARE PLAN: Palliative Care

This care plan must be reviewed monthly (or more often if required) and each action must be signed and dated

Patient's Issues and Objectives	Consultation Assessment and Plan	Signature	Date	Review Date
	10. Note any issues with the patient's dietary and fluid intake and the agreed plan of care to address this:			
	11. Note any issues with the patient's oral hygiene and the agreed plan of care to address this:			
	12. Note any issues with the patient's bladder or bowel function and the agreed plan of care to address this:			
	13. Record the patient's spiritual beliefs and the agreed plan of care:			
	14. Note and have regard for the wishes of the patient's family:			
	15. Monitor the patient's condition and liaise with the General Practitioner and healthcare professionals as necessary.			

Name	Patient/Relative Signature	Date

Copyright © 2020 Planning For Care Limited

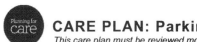

CARE PLAN: Parkinson's Disease

This care plan must be reviewed monthly (or more often if required) and each action must be signed and dated

Parkinson's disease is a degenerative disorder of the central nervous system. It results from the death of dopamine-containing cells in the substantia nigra, a region of the midbrain. The cause of cell-death is unknown. Early in the course of the disease, the most obvious symptoms are movement-related, including shaking, rigidity, slowness of movement and difficulty with walking and gait. Later, cognitive and behavioural problems may arise, with dementia commonly occurring in the advanced stages of the disease. Other symptoms include sensory, sleep and emotional problems.

Patient's Issues and Objectives	Consultation Assessment and Plan	Signature	Date	Review Date
Parkinson's Disease To maintain an optimal level of independence and lifestyle	1. Discuss the condition with the patient and, or relatives and agree the plan of care.			
	2. Note the patient's and, or relative's understanding of the condition and any concerns or anxieties they have:			
	3. Note the patient's past history of the condition if available:			
	4. Highlight symptoms of Parkinson's disease experienced: | SLOWNESS OF MOVEMENT | MUSCLE STIFFNESS | | RIGIDITY | TREMOR | BALANCE PROBLEMS | NERVE PAIN | CONSTIPATION | DYSPHAGIA | EXCESSIVE SALIVA | | SWALLOWING DIFFICULTY | WEIGHT LOSS |URINARY INCONTINENCE | NEEDING TO URINATE DURING THE NIGHT | | POSTURAL HYPOTENSION | DIZZINESS | EXCESSIVE SWEATING | LOSS OF SENSE OF SMELL | DAYTIME DOSING | | DEPRESSION | ANXIETY | DEMENTIA | HALLUCINATIONS | DELUSIONS |			
	5. Note the prescribed medication, dose and frequency:			
	6. Highlight any activities of daily living which are affected by Parkinson's disease: | RISING FROM BED | GOING TO BED | AFTER BEING IMMOBILE FOR PERIODS | GETTING UP FROM A CHAIR | | WASHING | DRESSING | UNDRESSING | CUTTING FOOD UP | EATING | DRINKING | GOING TO THE TOILET | | MOBILISING | ATTENDING ACTIVITIES |			
	7. Note in detail the daily routine and the agreed assistance required by the patient for the activities of daily living:			

Copyright © 2020 Planning For Care Limited

CARE PLAN: Parkinson's Disease

This care plan must be reviewed monthly (or more often if required) and each action must be signed and dated

Patient's Issues and Objectives	Consultation Assessment and Plan	Signature	Date	Review Date
	8. Note if the level of care required varies on a day to day basis due to changes in the patient's condition:			
	9. Note the agreed plan of care for the patient's mobility and periods of rest to prevent fatigue:			
	10. Highlight any specialised equipment that may assist the patient: | ANTI SPILLAGE CUP | ADAPTED CUTLERY | MECHANICAL HELPING HAND | NON SLIP MATS | PLATE GUARDS |			
	11. Encourage the patient to take warm baths and massage.			
	12. Monitor the patient's nutritional state and weight monthly or more frequently if required.			
	13. Administer the prescribed medication, monitor effects and liaise with the General Practitioner as necessary.			

Name	Patient/Relative Signature	Date

Copyright © 2020 Planning For Care Limited

CARE PLAN: Percutaneous Endoscopic Gastrostomy PEG Feed

This care plan must be reviewed monthly (or more often if required) and each action must be signed and dated

Percutaneous endoscopic gastrostomy, PEG, is an endoscopic medical procedure in which a tube, PEG tube, is passed into a patient's stomach through the abdominal wall, most commonly to provide a means of feeding when oral intake is not adequate. Neurological conditions are most commonly associated with such disability and constitute the most common indication for PEG. Many stroke sufferers, for example, are at risk of aspiration pneumonia due to poor control over the swallowing muscles. PEG feeding does not eliminate the risk of aspiration but it does reduce it.

Patient's Issues and Objectives	Consultation Assessment and Plan	Signature	Date	Review Date
Percutaneous endoscopic gastrostomy To maintain adequate nutrition and prevent any infection or complications of PEG feeding	1. Discuss the Peg feeding with the patient and, or relative and agree the plan of care.			
	2. Note the patient's and, or relative's understanding of this method of feeding and any concerns or anxieties they have:			
	3. Note the reason for having a PEG tube inserted:			
	4. Note how the patient is coping emotionally with this type of feeding and identify if they have any requests:			
	5. Note the prescribed feed and rate of administration:			
	6. Observe for signs of the patient aspirating, and any signs of discomfort.			
	7. Observe the PEG tube for any blockage, flush the PEG tube between meals with cooled boiled water.			
	8. The PEG tube site should be cleaned daily using normal saline and rotated 90 degrees each time it is cleaned.			
	9. Note the agreed plan of care for oral hygiene and any assistance required:			
	10. Weigh the patient on a monthly basis or more frequently as required and monitor their weight.			

Copyright © 2020 Planning For Care Limited

CARE PLAN: Percutaneous Endoscopic Gastrostomy PEG Feed

This care plan must be reviewed monthly (or more often if required) and each action must be signed and dated

Patient's Issues and Objectives	Consultation Assessment and Plan	Signature	Date	Review Date
	11. Liaise with the General Practitioner, dietician, and speech and language therapists as required.			

Name	Patient/Relative Signature	Date

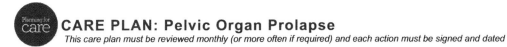

CARE PLAN: Pelvic Organ Prolapse
This care plan must be reviewed monthly (or more often if required) and each action must be signed and dated

Pelvic organ prolapse is the abnormal descent or herniation of the pelvic organs from their normal position in the pelvis. The pelvic structures that may be involved include the uterus, uterine prolapse, or vaginal apex, apical vaginal prolapse, anterior vagina, cystocele, or posterior vagina, rectocele. Many women who have had children may have some degree of prolapse when examined, however, most prolapses are not clinically bothersome without specific pelvic symptoms, and they may not require an intervention. The treatment of the prolapse depends on the severity of the symptoms, the severity of the prolapse, and the age and health of the patient. Treatment may not be necessary if the prolapse is mild to moderate and not causing any pain or discomfort.

Patient's Issues and Objectives	Consultation Assessment and Plan	Signature	Date	Review Date
Pelvic Organ Prolapse To promote effective management of the issue To maintain an optimal level of independence and lifestyle	**1. Discuss the condition with the patient and, or relative and agree the plan of care.**			
	2. Note the patient's and, or relative's understanding of the prolapse and any concerns or anxieties they have:			
	3. Note the past medical history of the prolapse, when it was diagnosed, and treatments prescribed:			
	4. Highlight the symptoms experienced by the patient: • A sensation of a bulge or something coming down or out of the vagina, which sometimes needs to be pushed back • Discomfort during sex • Problems passing urine, such as slow stream, • A feeling of not emptying the bladder fully, • Needing to urinate more often • Stress incontinence, leaking a small amount of urine when you cough, sneeze or exercise			
	5. Note any prescribed treatment where applicable:			
	6. Detail any issues the patient has with any activities of daily living, due to the prolapse, and the agreed plan to address them:			

Copyright © 2020 Planning For Care Limited

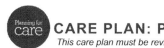

CARE PLAN: Pelvic Organ Prolapse

This care plan must be reviewed monthly (or more often if required) and each action must be signed and dated

Patient's Issues and Objectives	Consultation Assessment and Plan	Signature	Date	Review Date
	7. To avoid making the prolapse worse, it is important to encourage the patient to: • do regular pelvic floor exercises • maintaining a healthy weight • eat a high-fibre diet with plenty of fresh fruit, vegetables, and wholegrain bread and cereal to avoid constipation and straining when going to the toilet • avoid heavy lifting and standing up for long periods of time • stop smoking			
	8. Monitor the patient's prolapse and liaise with the General Practitioner as required.			

Name	Patient/Relative Signature	Date

Copyright © 2020 Planning For Care Limited

CARE PLAN: Pernicious Anaemia

This care plan must be reviewed monthly (or more often if required) and each action must be signed and dated

Pernicious, vitamin B12 or folate deficiency anaemia occurs when a lack of either of these vitamins affects the body's ability to produce fully functioning red blood cells. Red blood cells carry oxygen around the body. The cells of the body use the oxygen to break down sugar and fat, which then produces the body's energy, so if there is insufficient oxygen there is likely to be a lack of energy. Most people with vitamin B12 or folate deficiency anaemia have red blood cells, which are underdeveloped and larger than normal. Pernicious anaemia is an autoimmune condition, which affects the stomach. It causes the immune system to attack the cells in the stomach, which produce the intrinsic factor, which means it is unable to absorb vitamin B12. It is also possible to develop a vitamin B12 deficiency as a result of not getting enough vitamin B12 from diet such as a vegan diet may lack the intrinsic factor because it does not include eating meat.

Patient's Issues and Objectives	Consultation Assessment and Plan	Signature	Date	Review Date
Pernicious Anaemia To maintain haemoglobin within normal levels To identify and alleviate signs and symptoms of anaemia To prevent complications of anaemia To alleviate any concerns the patient may have	**1. Discuss the condition with the patient and, or relative and agree the plan of care.**			
	2. Note the patient's and, or relative's understanding of the condition and any concerns or anxieties they have:			
	3. Note when the patient was first diagnosed and any treatment they have received:			
	4. Highlight any of the following signs and symptoms of anaemia that the patient has experienced: | EXTREME TIREDNESS | LETHARGY LACK OF ENERGY | BREATHLESSNESS | FEELING FAINT | HEADACHES | | LOOKING PALE | RAPID PULSE | PALPITATIONS | DIZZINESS | LEG PAINS | TINNITUS | LOSS OF APETITE | | WEIGHT LOSS | YELLOW TINGE TO THE SKIN | SORE RED TONGUE | MOUTH ULCERS | PINS AND NEEDLES | | CHANGES IN WALKING AND MOVING AROUND | DISTURBED VISION | IRRITABLITY | DEPRESSION | DIARRHOEA | | REDUCED SENSE OF TASTE | NUMBNESS AND | TINGLING IN FEET AND HANDS | MUSCLE WEAKNESS |			
	5. Note any signs and symptoms which persist and the agreed plan of care to assist and support the patient:			
	6. Note any advice regarding the patient's diet:			

Copyright © 2020 Planning For Care Limited

CARE PLAN: Pernicious Anaemia

This care plan must be reviewed monthly (or more often if required) and each action must be signed and dated

Patient's Issues and Objectives	Consultation Assessment and Plan	Signature	Date	Review Date
	7. Note prescribed medication for pernicious anaemia, dose and frequency:			
	8. Obtain bloods and send to the laboratory for analysis annually or whenever requested by the patient's General Practitioner. Note the date taken:................................			
	9. Monitor the patient's condition and liaise with the General Practitioner as required.			

Name	Patient/Relative Signature	Date

CARE PLAN: Personal Hygiene

This care plan must be reviewed monthly (or more often if required) and each action must be signed and dated

Good personal hygiene helps prevent infection, cross infection and illness and it is very important for self esteem. Bathing, showering and washing displace dead skin cells and prevent irritations and rashes that would otherwise transform into infections. It is also extremely important to wash away waste materials that interfere with normal functioning of the skin.

Patient's Issues and Objectives	Consultation Assessment and Plan	Signature	Date	Review Date
Personal Hygiene To ensure a high standard of personal hygiene in accordance with the patient's choice	1. Discuss with the patient and, or relative any issues the patient has with maintaining their personal hygiene and identify where assistance would be beneficial.			
	2. Highlight the areas of the body the patient needs assistance with, when washing and drying: | FACE | EARS | NECK | CHEST | ABDOMEN | BACK | ARMS | HANDS | NAILS | FRONT OF LEGS | BACK OF LEGS | | FEET | GENITAL AREA | SACRAL AREA |..			
	3. Note if the level of assistance required varies from daily and the reason:			
	4. Highlight or detail where the patient likes to get washed: | ENSUITE TOILET | BATHROOM OF CHOICE | | BEDROOM WITH BASIN | IT VARIES:			
	5. Detail the agreed plan of care regarding assistance with personal hygiene, and preferences such as deodorant, perfume, aftershave:			
	6. Highlight any assistance required for the patient's nail care: | SELF CARE | ASSIST WITH CLEANING NAILS | | REMIND PATIENT TO CLEAN NAILS |...			
	7. Highlight the patient's preference: | FACE CLOTH | SPONGE |			
	8. Note how many towels the patient prefers when washing:			
	9. Highlight the assistance required for the patient's mouth care: | SELF CARE | NEEDS TO BE REMINDED | | NEEDS ASSISTANCE | VARIES DAILY |SPECIFY:			
	10. Highlight the assistance required for shaving and the preferred method: | NOT APPLICABLE | SELF CARE | | OWN ELECTRIC RAZOR | DISPOSABLE RAZOR | REQUIRES TO BE REMINDED | NEEDS ASSISTANCE | | VARIES DAILY |...			

Copyright © 2020 Planning For Care Limited

CARE PLAN: Personal Hygiene
This care plan must be reviewed monthly (or more often if required) and each action must be signed and dated

Patient's Issues and Objectives	Consultation Assessment and Plan	Signature	Date	Review Date
	11. Highlight any assistance required to care for the patient's hair: | SELF CARE | REMIND PATIENT TO BRUSH HAIR | ASSIST PATIENT TO BRUSH HAIR |................................			
	12. Highlight any assistance required for the patient's hearing aid: | DOES NOT REQUIRE ONE | SELF CARE | | REMIND TO PUT HEARING AID IN | ASSIST TO PUT HEARING AID IN AND TO REMOVE IT |.................................			
	13. Ensure the hearing aid is in good working order daily and note which ear requires it:			
	14. Highlight any assistance required for the patient's glasses: | DOES NOT NEED GLASSES | SELF CARE | | REMIND TO PUT GLASSES ON | REQUIRES ASSISTANCE CLEANING AND PUTTING GLASSES ON |....................			
	15. Highlight type of glasses: | READING | DISTANCE | BIFOCAL |			
	16. Note whether the patient prefers a bath or shower, how frequently and the preferred time(s):			
	17. Observe skin integrity daily and report any abnormalities to senior staff and record in the patient's notes.			
	....			

Name	Patient /Relative Signature	Date

Copyright © 2020 Planning For Care Limited

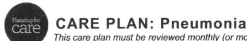

CARE PLAN: Pneumonia

This care plan must be reviewed monthly (or more often if required) and each action must be signed and date

Pneumonia is inflammation of the tissue in one or both lungs. It is usually a result of an infection, which causes the clusters of tiny air sacs in the lungs to become inflamed and fill up with fluid. The inflammation makes breathing more difficult and also causes a decrease in the absorption of oxygen. Other symptoms include a cough, which may be dry at first or productive with yellow, green, brownish or blood-stained phlegm. Other common symptoms include difficulty in breathing, which may be rapid and shallow, even at rest, a rapid heartbeat, fever, feeling generally unwell, sweating and shivering, loss of appetite, chest pain and an acute confused state. For people with other health conditions, pneumonia can be severe and may need to be treated in hospital, as there can be complications, some of which can be fatal, depending on their health and age. These include respiratory failure, when the lungs cannot take in enough oxygen, due to the air sacs filling with water, as well as lung abscesses and septicaemia.

Patient's Issues and Objectives	Consultation Assessment and Plan	Signature	Date	Review Date
Pneumonia To promote the healing process To prevent recurrence, and to reassure the patient	1. Discuss the condition with the patient and, or the relative and agree the plan of care.			
	2. Note the patient's and, or relative's understanding of the condition and any concerns or anxieties they have:			
	3. Note the patient's temperature, pulse, respirations, and blood pressure:			
	4. Highlight any symptoms experienced by the patient: | DIFFICULTY BREATHING | COUGHING UP YELLOW, GREEN, OR BROWN PHLEGM | RAPID HEARTBEAT | FEVER | | FEELING GENERALLY UNWELL | SWEATING | SHIVERING | LOSS OF APPETITE | CHEST PAIN WHEN BREATHING | | CHEST PAIN WHEN COUGHING | COUGHING UP BLOOD | HEADACHES | FATIGUE | NAUSEA | PAIN IN MUSCLES | | PAIN IN JOINTS | VOMITING | WHEEZING | CONFUSION |........................			
	5. If the patient has a productive cough, a sputum specimen should be sent to the laboratory for analysis. Note date sent:			
	6. Consult with General Practitioner for antibiotics and, or other medication.			
	7. Note the prescribed medication, dose and frequency:			
	8. Highlight the actions which form part of the agreed care plan for the patient: • encourage the patient to sit up in a chair for periods throughout the day • encourage the patient to be in an upright sitting position when in bed • encourage the patient to eat and drink adequate fluids			

Copyright © 2020 Planning For Care Limited

CARE PLAN: Pneumonia

This care plan must be reviewed monthly (or more often if required) and each action must be signed and date

Patient's Issues and Objectives	Consultation Assessment and Plan	Signature	Date	Review Date
	9. Note any additional plan of care required for the safety, adequate hydration, postural drainage, comfort and mental stimulation of the patient:			
	10. Monitor the patient's temperature, pulse, respirations, and blood pressure, daily or more frequently if required.			
	11. Monitor the patient for breathing difficulties, chest pain, and a productive cough.			
	12. Monitor the patient's condition liaising with the General Practitioner if there is no improvement by 3rd or 4th day.			
	....			

Name	Patient/Relative Signature	Date

CARE PLAN: Post Fracture

This care plan must be reviewed monthly (or more often if required) and each action must be signed and date

A fracture is a break in bone or cartilage, although it is usually the result of trauma, it can be caused by an acquired disease of bone such as osteoporosis. The aim of treatment is to assist the bone to recover fully in strength, movement and sensitivity. Some complicated fractures may need surgery or surgical traction. Following diagnosis of the fracture, the treatment is to realign the bone ends and immobilise the fracture by external splints or internal fixing of the bone, or both for best results. When a bone fractures there's usually a lot of soft tissue and structure damage and the treatment of immobilising the area in plaster or surgically can lead to stiffness and considerable weakness. This may even affect joints that do not seem related to the break. A fractured shoulder may result in a very stiff elbow or wrist due to keeping the shoulder in a sling for a few weeks.

Patient's Issues and Objectives	Consultation Assessment and Plan	Signature	Date	Review Date
Return from hospital Post Fracture **Assess the patient's mobility following discharge and offer all assistance and aids required**	1. Discuss the condition with the patient and, or relative and agree the plan of care.			
	2. Note the patient's and, or relative's understanding of the condition and any concerns or anxieties they have:			
	3. Note the type of fracture and the area affected:			
	4. Note the treatment received:			
	5. Note any prescribed analgesia, the frequency and dose:			
	6. Note in detail the assistance the patient requires due to the fracture:			
	7. Discuss and agree the rest and rehabilitation plan with the patient and, or relative. Rehabilitation plan: .... Rest plan:			

Copyright © 2020 Planning For Care Limited

CARE PLAN: Post Fracture

This care plan must be reviewed monthly (or more often if required) and each action must be signed and date

Patient's Issues and Objectives	Consultation Assessment and Plan	Signature	Date	Review Date
	8. Identify any issues affecting the patient's rehabilitation plan:			
	9. Note any additional agreed plan of care:			
	10. Liaise with the patient's General Practitioner as necessary.			

Name	Patient/Relative Signature	Date

Copyright © 2020 Planning For Care Limited

CARE PLAN: Pressure Area Care

This care plan must be reviewed monthly (or more often if required) and each action must be signed and dated

Relief of pressure or position changes are key to pressure sore prevention. These changes need to be frequent, repositioning needs to avoid stress on the skin, and body positions need to minimize the risk of pressure on vulnerable areas. Other strategies include skin care, regular skin inspections and good nutrition. As little as two hours of sustained pressure can trigger skin damage. Skin damage can also be exacerbated by friction and moisture. The surface damage is just the tip of the iceberg, the real damage lies beneath the surface of the skin.

Patient's Issues and Objectives	Consultation Assessment and Plan	Signature	Date	Review Date
High risk of developing a pressure sore **To relieve pressure and maintain skin integrity**	1. Discuss with the patient and, or relative the Waterlow assessment score, indicating a high risk of skin breakdown and agree the plan of care.			
	2. Note the patient's and, or relative's understanding of the risk and any concerns or anxieties they have:			
	3. Highlight any contributing factors experienced by the patient which increase the risk of skin breakdown: | BED REST | INCONTINENCE | DIABETES | ANAEMIA | IMMOBILITY | CARDIAC FAILURE | POOR NUTRITION | OEDEMA | | MEDICATION |			
	4. Note the agreed plan to address and improve the contributing factors, where possible:			
	5. Note the type of pressure relieving equipment required for the patient's bed and chair:			
	6. Note or highlight the agreed plan of care to relieve or alleviate pressure: | COMMENCE CHANGE OF POSITION CHART | ENCOURAGE INTERMITTENT BED REST | | ENCOURAGE OR HELP THE PATIENT TO STAND UP AT VARIOUS INTERVALS THROUGHOUT THE DAY | **Specify plan of care:**			

Copyright © 2020 Planning For Care Limited

CARE PLAN: Pressure Area Care

This care plan must be reviewed monthly (or more often if required) and each action must be signed and dated

Patient's Issues and Objectives	Consultation Assessment and Plan	Signature	Date	Review Date
	7. Review the risk assessment monthly.			

Name	Patient/Relative Signature	Date

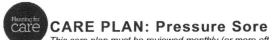

CARE PLAN: Pressure Sore

This care plan must be reviewed monthly (or more often if required) and each action must be signed and dated

Pressure sores or bed sores are painful skin ulcers that form when constant pressure on a part of the body shuts down the blood vessels feeding that area of skin. The resulting damage first appears on the skin surface as a red or dark patch. As the pressure sore progresses, the skin will break down to form blisters, dead skin, and ultimately infect underlying tissues, bones and joints. As little as two hours of sustained pressure can trigger skin damage. Skin damage can also be exacerbated by friction and moisture. The surface damage is just the tip of the iceberg; the real damage lies beneath the surface of the skin.

Patient's Issues and Objectives	Consultation Assessment and Plan	Signature	Date	Review Date
Pressure Sore To heal the pressure sore and maintain skin integrity	1. Discuss the issue with the patient and, or relative and agree the plan of care.			
	2. Note the patient's and, or relative's understanding of the issue and any concerns or anxieties they have:			
	3. Highlight any factors which affect the patient and could delay healing: | INCONTINENCE | DIABETES | ANAEMIA | IMMOBILITY | CARDIAC FAILURE | OEDEMA | INFECTION | MEDICATION | | POOR NUTRITION |			
	4. Note the agreed plan of care to address the identified factors where possible:			
	5. Specify the location of the patient's pressure sore:			
	6. Complete a formal wound assessment, noting the size of wound, the type of wound, any exudate present, the depth of the wound and the condition of the surrounding skin.			
	7. Consult with the patient's General Practitioner to assess the wound and note the prescribed treatment in the wound treatment plan.			
	8. Ensure the wound assessment chart and treatment plan is completed at each dressing change.			
	9. Regularly explain all treatment and progress to the patient.			
	10. Note the prescribed plan of treatment for the wound:			

Copyright © 2020 Planning For Care Limited

CARE PLAN: Pressure Sore

This care plan must be reviewed monthly (or more often if required) and each action must be signed and dated

Patient's Issues and Objectives	Consultation Assessment and Plan	Signature	Date	Review Date
	11. Note the agreed plan of care to minimise and alleviate pressure to the affected area:			
	12. Note the type of pressure relieving mattress and cushion:			
	13. Note the assistance required for frequent changes of position. During the day: During the night:			
	14. Note the prescribed treatment for pain management:			
	15. Monitor the wound and liaise with the General Practitioner and, or tissue viability nurse if necessary.			

Name	Patient/Relative Signature	Date

Copyright © 2020 Planning For Care Limited

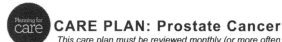

CARE PLAN: Prostate Cancer

This care plan must be reviewed monthly (or more often if required) and each action must be signed and dated

Prostate cancer usually develops slowly, so there may be no signs or symptoms for many years. Symptoms often only become apparent when the prostate is large enough to affect the urethra, the tube that carries urine from the bladder to the penis. This may cause an increased need to urinate, straining while urinating and a feeling that the bladder has not fully emptied. If the cancer spreads to other parts of the body, typically the bones, it often cannot be cured and treatment is focused on prolonging life and relieving the symptoms. If the cancer is at an early stage and not causing symptoms, a policy of carefully monitoring the condition may be adopted. Some cases of prostate cancer can be cured if treated in the early stages. Treatments can include surgically removing the prostate, radiotherapy and hormone therapy. All treatments carry the risk of side effects, including erectile dysfunction and urinary incontinence, and for this reason, many men choose to delay treatment until there is a risk the cancer might spread.

Patient's Issues and Objectives	Consultation Assessment and Plan	Signature	Date	Review Date
Prostate Cancer To promote effective management of the condition To maintain an optimal level of independence and lifestyle	**1. Discuss the condition with the patient and, or relative and agree the plan of care.**			
	2. Note the patient's and, or relative's understanding of the condition and any concerns or anxieties they have:			
	3. Highlight the diagnosed stage of the prostate cancer, where known: • Stage I. Early cancer that is confined to a small area of the prostate, cancer cells are not considered aggressive • Stage II. Cancer at this stage may still be small, but may be considered aggressive, or cancer that is stage II may be larger and may have grown to involve both sides of the prostate gland • Stage III. The cancer has spread beyond the prostate to the seminal vesicles or other nearby tissues • Stage IV. The cancer has grown to invade nearby organs, the bladder, lymph nodes, bones, lungs or other organs			
	4. Note when the patient was diagnosed as having prostate cancer, and any treatment received:			
	5. Highlight any symptoms experienced by the patient: | DIFFICULTY STARTING TO URINATE | BLOOD IN URINE | | FATIGUE | FLOW OF URINE STOPS AND STARTS | STRAINS TO PASSS URINE | URGENT URGE TO URINATE | | URINATES FREQUENTLY | NEEDS TO URINATE FREQUENTLY DURING THE NIGHT | INCONTINENT OF URINE | | CANNOT FULLY EMPTY THE BLADDER | SPECIFY:			
	6. Note the agreed plan of care to assist the patient with any symptoms they are experiencing:			

Copyright © 2020 Planning For Care Limited

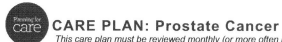

CARE PLAN: Prostate Cancer

This care plan must be reviewed monthly (or more often if required) and each action must be signed and dated

Patient's Issues and Objectives	Consultation Assessment and Plan	Signature	Date	Review Date
	7. Ensure a Care Plan is completed for any issues or symptoms experienced as a result of the cancer or treatment.			
	8. Note the prescribed medication, dosage and frequency if applicable:			
	9. Monitor the patient's urinary output, observe for any signs of a urinary tract infection, which can include: | A NEED TO URINATE MORE FREQUENTLY | CONSTANT DULL PAIN IN PUBIC REGION | PAIN WHEN URINATING | | CLOUDY URINE | BLOOD IN URINE | FOUL SMELLING URINE | BACK PAIN | GENERALLY FEELING UNWELL |			
	10. Observe the patient for symptoms of acute urinary retention, seek urgent medical assistance if they have: | A SUDDEN INABILITY TO PASS URINE | SEVERE LOWER ABDOMINAL PAIN | SWELLING OF THE BLADDER |			

Name	Patient/Relative Signature	Date

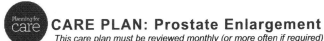

CARE PLAN: Prostate Enlargement

This care plan must be reviewed monthly (or more often if required) and each action must be signed and dated

Prostate enlargement, also known as benign prostatic hyperplasia, is a common condition that affects older men. The prostate is a small gland found in men, located between the penis and bladder. If the prostate becomes enlarged, it can place pressure on the bladder and urethra, the tube through which urine passes. This can cause a difficulty starting urination, a frequent need to urinate, or a difficulty fully emptying the bladder. These symptoms can range from mild to severe. Men with prostate enlargement do not have a higher risk of prostate cancer compared to men without an enlarged prostate. Prostate enlargement is a common condition associated with ageing. Around 60% of men, aged 60 or over have some degree of prostate enlargement. The cause is unknown, but it may be due to changes in hormone levels in a man's body due to ageing. Complications can include urinary tract infections, bladder stones, kidney damage and acute urinary retention which is a medical emergency requiring immediate action.

Patient's Issues and Objectives	Consultation Assessment and Plan	Signature	Date	Review Date
Prostate Enlargement To promote effective management of the condition To maintain an optimal level of independence and lifestyle	1. Discuss the condition with the patient and, or relative and agree the plan of care.			
	2. Note the patient's and, or relative's understanding of the condition and any concerns or anxieties they have:			
	3. Note the past medical history of prostate enlargement, when it was diagnosed and any treatment received:			
	4. Highlight the symptoms experienced by the patient: | DIFFICULTY IN STARTING TO URINATE | FLOW OF URINE STOPS AND STARTS | STRAINS TO PASSS URINE | | URINATES FREQUENTLY | NEEDS TO URINATE FREQUENTLY DURING THE NIGHT | INCONTINENT OF URINE | | URGENT URGE TO URINATE | CANNOT FULLY EMPTY THE BLADDER | BLOOD IN THE URINE | SPECIFY:			
	5. Note the prescribed medication, dosage and frequency if applicable:			
	6. Note in detail the assistance the patient requires due to the symptoms experienced:			

Copyright © 2020 Planning For Care Limited

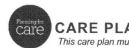

CARE PLAN: Prostate Enlargement

This care plan must be reviewed monthly (or more often if required) and each action must be signed and dated

Patient's Issues and Objectives	Consultation Assessment and Plan	Signature	Date	Review Date
	7. Consider and highlight any lifestyle changes which may help to manage or alleviate the symptoms: • avoid drinking one or two hours before going to bed • avoid drinking alcohol or caffeine as this can irritate the bladder			
	8. Monitor the patient's urinary output, observe any signs of a urinary tract infection, which can include: | A NEED TO URINATE MORE FREQUENTLY | CONSTANT DULL PAIN IN PUBIC REGION | PAIN WHEN URINATING | | CLOUDY URINE | BLOOD IN URINE | FOUL SMELLING URINE| BACK PAIN | GENERALLY FEELING UNWELL |			
	9. Liaise with the patient's General Practitioner immediately if the patient shows signs of a urinary tract infection.			
	10. Observe the patient for symptoms of acute urinary retention and seek urgent medical assistance if: • there is the sudden inability to pass urine • the patient has severe lower abdominal pain • there is swelling of the bladder			
	....			

Name	Patient/Relative Signature	Date

Copyright © 2020 Planning For Care Limited

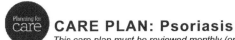

CARE PLAN: Psoriasis

This care plan must be reviewed monthly (or more often if required) and each action must be signed and dated

Psoriasis occurs when the skin cells replace themselves too quickly. It usually takes up to 28 days for newly formed skin cells to rise to the surface of the skin and separate from healthy tissue, but in psoriasis it takes just two to six days. There are many different types, but the most common is chronic plaque psoriasis. Psoriasis usually appears as red, scaly, crusty patches that reveal fine silver scales when scraped or scratched. These patches may itch and feel sore and uncomfortable. Psoriasis is most common on the knees, elbows and scalp, but can appear anywhere on the body. In some forms the nails or joints are affected. The cause of psoriasis is unknown but many things are thought to trigger the condition including a skin injury, sore throat or chest infection, alcohol, certain drug treatments, sunburn and stress.

Patient's Issues and Objectives	Consultation Assessment and Plan	Signature	Date	Review Date
Psoriasis Promotion and maintenance of healthy skin	1. Discuss the condition with the patient and, or relative and agree the plan of care.			
	2. Note the patient's and, or relative's understanding of the condition and any concerns or anxieties they have:			
	3. Identify the area(s) affected with psoriasis:			
	4. Highlight and discuss with the patient and, or relatives any possible contributing factors: | TRAUMA OR INJURY TO THE SKIN | EXCESSIVE ALCOHOL | SMOKING | STRESS | HORMONAL CHANGES | | MEDICINES SUCH AS LITHIUM, IBUPROFEN ACE INHIBITORS | THROAT INFECTION | IMMUNE DISORDERS | HIV |			
	5. Note the agreed plan to address and improve the contributing factors, where possible:			
	6. Consult with the patient's General Practitioner.			
	7. Note the prescribed medication and treatment regime:			
	8. Identify any issues with the application of creams:			

Copyright © 2020 Planning For Care Limited

CARE PLAN: Psoriasis

This care plan must be reviewed monthly (or more often if required) and each action must be signed and dated

Patient's Issues and Objectives	Consultation Assessment and Plan	Signature	Date	Review Date
	9. Monitor the effectiveness of the treatment and condition.			
	10. Identify any psychological issues the patient has due to the condition:			
	11. Liaise with the patient's General Practitioner as necessary.			

Name	Patient/Relative Signature	Date

Copyright © 2020 Planning For Care Limited

CARE PLAN: Pulmonary Embolism

This care plan must be reviewed monthly (or more often if required) and each action must be signed and dated

A pulmonary embolism is a blood clot in the pulmonary artery, which is the blood vessel that transports blood from the heart to the lungs. It is a serious and potentially life-threatening condition as it can prevent the blood from reaching the lungs. When the blood leaves the heart, it is low in oxygen and needs to reach the lungs to pick up oxygen. Pulmonary embolisms often occur when part or all of a blood clot, a Deep Vein Thrombosis, travels from one of the deep veins in the legs to the lungs. The signs and symptoms of a pulmonary embolism can sometimes be difficult to recognise because they can vary between individuals. The main symptoms include chest pain, a sharp stabbing pain that may be worse when breathing in, shortness of breath which can come on suddenly or develop gradually and coughing which may include coughing up blood or mucous containing blood, anxiety, feeling faint or dizzy, or sudden collapse.

Patient's Issues and Objectives	Consultation Assessment and Plan	Signature	Date	Review Date
Pulmonary Embolism To promote the healing process, to prevent recurrence, and to reassure the patient	1. Discuss the condition with the patient and, or the relative and agree the plan of care.			
	2. Note the patient's and, or relative's understanding of the condition and any concerns or anxieties they have:			
	3. Record the patient's temperature, pulse, respirations, and blood pressure:			
	4. Highlight any symptoms experienced by the patient: | CHEST PAIN | BREATHLESSNESS | DRY COUGH | COUGHING UP BLOOD | BLOOD STAINED MUCOUS | DIZZINESS | | FEELING FAINT | FAINTING | SPECIFY:			
	5. Note the prescribed medication and anticoagulant treatment regime:			
	6. Note the agreed plan of care:			
	7. Monitor the patient's temperature, pulse, respirations, and blood pressure, daily or more frequently if required.			
	8. If Warfarin is prescribed advise the patient to avoid taking any cranberry juice, cranberries, or products containing cranberries as it affects the warfarin therapy and ensure a warfarin care plan is completed.			

Copyright © 2020 Planning For Care Limited

CARE PLAN: Pulmonary Embolism

This care plan must be reviewed monthly (or more often if required) and each action must be signed and dated

Patient's Issues and Objectives	Consultation Assessment and Plan	Signature	Date	Review Date
	9. Monitor for signs and symptoms of complications such as chest pain or sudden collapse as this indicates a medical emergency.			
	10. Liaise with the patient's General Practitioner as required.			

Name	Patient/Relative Signature	Date

Copyright © 2020 Planning For Care Limited

CARE PLAN: Recreation

This care plan must be reviewed monthly (or more often if required) and each action must be signed and dated

Being involved in meaningful leisure activities often leads to improved self esteem, self worth, recognition, friendships, enjoyment, sense of belonging, improved physical health, and, or independence, all of which enhance the quality of life and contribute to well being. There is compelling evidence that a good diet, physical exercise, and mental stimulation all help prevent age-related cognitive decline and reduce the risk of mild cognitive impairment and Alzheimer's.

Patient's Issues and Objectives	Consultation Assessment and Plan	Signature	Date	Review Date
Recreation **To encourage and plan meaningful individualised leisure activities**	**1. Discuss with the patient and or relative all present, past and potential interests and detail them:**			
	2. Highlight any activity the patient is or may be interested in: | ART | MUSIC | WALKING | READING | CURRENT AFFAIRS | NEWS | REMINISCENCE | DEBATING | COMPUTING | | TELEVISION | VIDEOS | AROMATHERAPY | BEAUTY TREATMENTS | BUS OUTINGS | CARPET BOWLS | BINGO | | CARD GAMES | CHURCH SERVICES | COMMUNION | | CONCERTS | DOMINOES | EXERCISE CLASS | GARDENING | | KNITTING | MUSIC AND MOVEMENT | QUIZ GAMES | SINGALONGS | SKITTLES | TABLE GAMES | MEDITATION | OTHER:..			
	3. Note the agreed plan for the patient to be involved in recreational or leisure activities:			
	4. Note any unfulfilled life goals and any unfulfilled aspirations:			

Copyright © 2020 Planning For Care Limited

CARE PLAN: Recreation

This care plan must be reviewed monthly (or more often if required) and each action must be signed and dated

Patient's Issues and Objectives	Consultation Assessment and Plan	Signature	Date	Review Date
	5. Note where possible, the agreed plan to achieve any unfulfilled goals:			

Name	Patient/Relative Signature	Date

Copyright © 2020 Planning For Care Limited

CARE PLAN: Rheumatoid Arthritis

This care plan must be reviewed monthly (or more often if required) and each action must be signed and date

Rheumatoid arthritis is an autoimmune disease where the body's defence mechanisms go into action when there is no threat. The immune system attacks the joints and sometimes other parts of the body. It is not yet known why the immune system acts in this way in some people. The joints become inflamed, particularly the synovial membrane, the tendon sheaths, the fluid that allows muscles and tendons to move smoothly over one another. Inflammation sometimes becomes far worse, a flare up, when the joints become warm and red as blood flow to the area increases. The synovial membrane produces extra fluid, causing swelling and a stretching of the ligaments around the joint. The result is a stiff, swollen and painful joint. Treating inflammation quickly is vital because once joint damage has occurred it cannot be reversed.

Patient's Issues and Objectives	Consultation Assessment and Plan	Signature	Date	Review Date
Rheumatoid Arthritis To minimise pain and discomfort to promote effective management of the condition To maintain an optimal level of independence and lifestyle	1. Discuss the condition with the patient and, or relative and agree the plan of care.			
	2. Note the patient's and, or relative's understanding of the condition and any concerns or anxieties they have:			
	3. Note the past medical history of rheumatoid arthritis, when it was diagnosed and any treatments prescribed:			
	4. Note the areas affected:			
	5. Highlight symptoms evident or experienced by the patient: | JOINT PAIN | THROBBING PAIN | ACHING PAIN | JOINT STIFFNESS | SWELLING | REDNESS AROUND JOINTS | | JOINTS HOT AND TENDER TO TOUCH | FIRM SWELLINGS AROUND THE JOINTS | FATIGUE | FEVER | SWEATING | | POOR APPETITE | WEIGHT LOSS | DRY EYES | CHEST PAIN |			
	6. Highlight the activities of daily living the patient has issues with, due to having rheumatoid arthritis: | GETTING UP IN THE MORNING | DRESSING | EATING AND DRINKING | INSOMNIA DUE TO PAIN | MOBILITY | | GOING TO THE TOILET DUE TO REDUCED MOBILITY | CONSTIPATION DUE TO ANALGESIA | GOING TO BED | | SOCIALISING |			
	7. Note the agreed plan of care to address any activities of daily living the patient has issues with:			

Copyright © 2020 Planning For Care Limited

CARE PLAN: Rheumatoid Arthritis

This care plan must be reviewed monthly (or more often if required) and each action must be signed and date

Patient's Issues and Objectives	Consultation Assessment and Plan	Signature	Date	Review Date
	8. Note the prescribed medication, the dose and frequency:			
	9. Monitor the patient's condition and consult with General Practitioner as necessary.			

Name	Patient/Relative Signature	Date

CARE PLAN: Schizophrenia

This care plan must be reviewed monthly (or more often if required) and each action must be signed and dated

Schizophrenia is a long-term mental health condition which can cause a range of different psychological symptoms, including hallucinations, hearing or seeing things that do not exist, delusions, unusual beliefs which are not based on reality, muddled thoughts based on hallucinations or delusions, changes in behavior, a lack of interest in things, difficulty concentrating. Schizophrenia is often described as a psychotic illness, which means that the person with schizophrenia, may not be able to distinguish their own thoughts and ideas from reality. For some these experiences or beliefs can start happening quite suddenly, but for others they can occur more gradually. The person with schizophrenia may become upset, anxious, confused and suspicious of other people, particularly anyone who doesn't agree with their perceptions.

Patient's Issues and Objectives	Consultation Assessment and Plan	Signature	Date	Review Date
Schizophrenia To support the patient and manage the patient's symptoms to maximise their general well-being	1. Discuss the condition with the patient and, or relative and agree the plan of care.			
	2. Note the patient's and, or relative's understanding of the condition and any concerns or anxieties they have:			
	3. Note the patients past medical history of schizophrenia, how it affects the patient and the treatment prescribed:			
	5. Highlight any of the following "positive" signs and symptoms of schizophrenia experienced by the patient: | HALLUCINATIONS | DELUSIONS | THOUGHT DISORDER | HEARING VOICES | CONFUSED THOUGHTS | AGITATION | | SHOUTING | SWEARING |..			
	6. Highlight any of the following "negative" signs and symptoms of schizophrenia experienced by the patient: | SOCIAL WITHDRAWAL | POOR PERSONAL HYGIENE | LACK OF MOTIVATION | LACK OF CONCENTRATION | | AGRAPHOBIA |..			
	7. Detail what the patient experiences during a relapse in their condition or during a psychotic episode:			
	8. Note the agreed treatment plan:			

Copyright © 2020 Planning For Care Limited

CARE PLAN: Schizophrenia

This care plan must be reviewed monthly (or more often if required) and each action must be signed and dated

Patient's Issues and Objectives	Consultation Assessment and Plan	Signature	Date	Review Date
	9. Note and record the prescribed medication, dose and frequency if applicable:			
	10. Encourage the patient to express his or her feelings and thoughts and listen attentively.			
	11. Identify any issues the patient has with safety:			
	12. Monitor the patient's condition and liaise with the General Practitioner or Psychiatrist as required.			

Name	Patient/Relative Signature	Date

Copyright © 2020 Planning For Care Limited

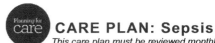

CARE PLAN: Sepsis

This care plan must be reviewed monthly (or more often if required) and each action must be signed and dated

Sepsis is a common and potentially life-threatening condition triggered by an infection. In sepsis, the body's immune system goes into overdrive, setting off a series of reactions including widespread inflammation, swelling and blood clotting. This can lead to a significant decrease in blood pressure, which can mean the blood supply to vital organs such as the brain, heart and kidneys is reduced. If not treated quickly, sepsis can eventually lead to multiple organ failure and death. The most common sites of infection leading to sepsis are the lungs, urinary tract, abdomen, and pelvis. As a result of problems with vital organs, people with severe sepsis or septic shock are likely to be very ill and up to four in every ten people with the condition will die. However, if identified and treated quickly, sepsis is treatable.

Patient's Issues and Objectives	Consultation Assessment and Plan	Signature	Date	Review Date
Sepsis Treat the infection and reduce risk of infection re-occurring	1. Discuss the condition with the patient and, or relatives and agree plan of care.			
	2. Note any concerns or anxieties the patient and, or the relatives have:			
	3. Note any history of previous infections:			
	4. Highlight which of the following infections, if known, the patient has been suffering from: | LUNG INFECTION | PNEUMONIA | APPENDICITIS | PERITONITIS | URINARY TRACT INFECTION | CHOLECYSTITIS | | CHOLANGITIS | KIDNEY INFECTION | CELLULITIS | POST SURGERY INFECTION | MENINGITIS | ENCEPHALITIS | | FLU | OTHER			
	5. Highlight which of the following signs and symptoms the patient is experiencing: | HIGH TEMPERATURE | FEVER | CHILLS | SHIVERING | FAST PULSE | FAST BREATHING |............................			
	6. Consult with the General Practitioner and detail the treatment advised:			
	7. Note the prescribed medication, dose and frequency:			

Copyright © 2020 Planning For Care Limited

CARE PLAN: Sepsis

This care plan must be reviewed monthly (or more often if required) and each action must be signed and dated

Patient's Issues and Objectives	Consultation Assessment and Plan	Signature	Date	Review Date
	8. Detail the agreed plan of care and assistance the patient requires:			
	9. Observe for any symptoms of septic shock which can include the following, seek immediate medical assistance:			
	| DROP IN BLOOD PRESSURE | SUDDEN FEELING OF WEAKNESS | FEELING DIZZY | LOSS OF CONSCIOUSNESS |			
	| VOMITING | NAUSEA | CONFUSION | DISORIENTATION | DIARRHOEA | COLD | CLAMMY | SLURRED SPEECH |			
	| SEVERE MUSCLE PAIN | SEVERE BREATHLESSNESS | DECREASED URINARY OUTPUT | MOTTLED SKIN |			

Name	Resident/Relative Signature	Date

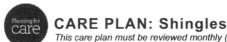

CARE PLAN: Shingles
This care plan must be reviewed monthly (or more often if required) and each action must be signed and dated

Shingles is an infection of a nerve and the area of the skin around it. It is caused by the herpes varicella-zoster virus, which also causes chickenpox. It usually affects a specific area on either the left or the right side of the body. There are three main stages, first, pain is felt in a localised area of the head, back or side, then a rash, blisters and flu-like symptoms occur, finally, the blisters erupt and pain increases which can lead to Post-Herpetic Neuralgia. If treatment is started within the first three days, there is a lower chance of complications such as post herpetic neuralgic pain. If a person has had chickenpox the virus remains in their body. This can re-emerge as shingles if their body defences or immunities are low. It is infectious only to people who have not had chickenpox and are therefore not immune to the virus. They would develop chickenpox, not shingles. The virus is not spread through sneezing, coughing or casual contact.

Patient's Issues and Objectives	Consultation Assessment and Plan	Signature	Date	Review Date
Shingles To effectively promote recovery and minimise any pain. To alleviate any concerns the patient may have and to prevent cross infection or contamination.	1. Reassure the patient and or relative, explain the condition and agree the plan of care.			
	2. Explain that shingles is contagious and good hand washing techniques are essential. It can be spread to anyone who has not had chickenpox and does not have immunity to the virus, they can develop chickenpox. Shingles is spread by the fluid from the blisters, or bedding, or towels which have been in contact with the fluid. Shingles rash is contagious until all blisters have scabbed and are dry, usually 5 to 7 days after the symptoms start.			
	3. Record any concerns or anxieties the patient or the relative has:			
	4. Specify the area(s) where shingles is evident:			
	5. Highlight any signs and symptoms experienced by the patient: | BURNING, TINGLING OR NUMBNESS OF THE SKIN | ITCHY SKIN | DULL PAIN | BURNING SENSATION | FEVER | | GENERALLY UNWELL | LOCALISED BAND OF PAIN | RASH USUALLY ON ONE SIDE OF THE BODY | BLISTERS | | SHARP STABBING PAINS | SCABS | HEADACHE | ………………			
	6. Note the prescribed treatment including analgesia:			
	7. Note the date treatment commenced:			
	8. Detail any issues the patient has with the activities of daily living, due to the condition, and the agreed plan to address them:			

Copyright © 2020 Planning For Care Limited

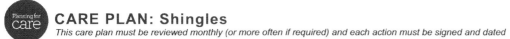

CARE PLAN: Shingles
This care plan must be reviewed monthly (or more often if required) and each action must be signed and dated

Patient's Issues and Objectives	Consultation Assessment and Plan	Signature	Date	Review Date
	9. If the face or head area, is affected, it may be advisable for the patient to avoid contact with others until the infectious stage is over and the blisters have crusted. Highlight the patient's preference for mental stimulation: | TELEVISION | DVDS | RADIO MUSIC | RADIO TALK SHOWS | READING | CROSSWORDS |………………………………			
	10. Inform all staff of the fact the patient has this infection and the importance of good hand washing techniques.			
	11. Ensure gloves and aprons are worn when working with the patient.			
	12. Ensure that clothing or bedding with bodily discharge is put into an alginate bag prior to laundering.			
	13. Liaise with the patient's General Practitioner as necessary.			

Name	Patient/Relative Signature	Date

Copyright © 2020 Planning For Care Limited

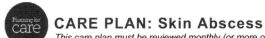

CARE PLAN: Skin Abscess

This care plan must be reviewed monthly (or more often if required) and each action must be signed and dated

An abscess is a painful collection of pus, usually caused by a bacterial infection, which can develop anywhere in the body. A skin abscess develops under the skin and often appears as a swollen, pus-filled lump under the surface of the skin. There may also be other symptoms of an infection, such as a high temperature, fever or chill. When bacteria enter the body, the immune system sends infection-fighting white blood cells to the affected area. As the white blood cells attack the bacteria, some nearby tissue dies, creating a hole which then fills with pus to form an abscess. The pus contains a mixture of dead tissue, white blood cells and bacteria. A small skin abscess may drain naturally, or simply shrink, dry up and disappear without any treatment. However, larger abscesses may need to be treated with antibiotics to clear the infection, and the pus may need to be drained. This will usually be done either by inserting a needle through the skin or by making a small incision in the skin over the abscess.

Patient's Issues and Objectives	Consultation Assessment and Plan	Signature	Date	Review Date
Skin Abscess **To treat the infection** **Promotion and maintenance of healthy skin**	1. Discuss the abscess with the patient and, or relative and agree the plan of care.			
	2. Note the patient's and, or the relative's understanding of the condition and any concerns or anxieties they have:			
	3. Detail the patient's past history of skin abscess:			
	4. Identify the area affected:			
	5. Highlight symptoms experienced by the patient: | TENDERNESS IN AFFECTED AREA | PAIN IN AFFECTED AREA | | RED AREA | HARD SWELLING UNDER THE SKIN | SWOLLEN PUS-FILLED SPOT | HIGH TEMPERATURE | | GENERALLY FEELING UNWELL |............			
	6. Note the prescribed medication and treatment regime:			
	7. Complete a wound assessment chart as necessary and update as necessary.			
	8. Liaise with the patient's General Practitioner as required.			

Copyright © 2020 Planning For Care Limited

CARE PLAN: Skin Abscess

This care plan must be reviewed monthly (or more often if required) and each action must be signed and dated

Patient's Issues and Objectives	Consultation Assessment and Plan	Signature	Date	Review Date

Name	Patient/Relative Signature	Date

Copyright © 2020 Planning For Care Limited

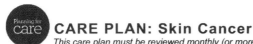

CARE PLAN: Skin Cancer

This care plan must be reviewed monthly (or more often if required) and each action must be signed and dated

Skin cancer is the abnormal growth of skin cells, which most often develops on skin exposed to the sun, but it can also occur on areas of the skin which is not ordinarily exposed to sunlight. There are three major types of skin cancer, basal cell carcinoma, squamous cell carcinoma and non-melanoma. Basal cell carcinoma usually occurs in sun-exposed areas of the body. Most often, squamous cell carcinoma occurs on sun-exposed areas of the body although, people with darker skin are more likely to develop squamous cell carcinoma on areas which are not often exposed to the sun. Melanoma can develop anywhere on the body, in otherwise normal skin or in an existing mole that becomes cancerous. Early detection of skin cancer gives the greatest chance for successful skin cancer treatment.

Patient's Issues and Objectives	Consultation Assessment and Plan	Signature	Date	Review Date
Skin Cancer Promotion and maintenance of healthy skin	1. Discuss the condition with the patient and, or relative and agree the plan of care.			
	2. Note the patient's and, or relative's understanding of the condition and any concerns or anxieties they have:			
	3. Detail the patient's past history, the type of skin cancer and any treatment received:			
	4. Identify the area(s) affected by skin cancer:			
	5. Detail the dimensions of the area of skin affected:			
	6. Detail the description and appearance of the skin cancer and note any associated symptoms experienced:			
	7. Note any prescribed treatment regime where applicable:			
	8. Identify any issues with the application of creams or treatment regime:			

Copyright © 2020 Planning For Care Limited

CARE PLAN: Skin Cancer

This care plan must be reviewed monthly (or more often if required) and each action must be signed and dated

Patient's Issues and Objectives	Consultation Assessment and Plan	Signature	Date	Review Date
	9. Liaise with the patient's General Practitioner or dermatologist or consultant as necessary.			

Name	Patient/Relative Signature	Date

Copyright © 2020 Planning For Care Limited

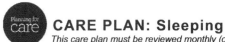

CARE PLAN: Sleeping

This care plan must be reviewed monthly (or more often if required) and each action must be signed and dated

Sleep is important for the body's rejuvenation. Sleep allows the body to restore tissues, energy levels and recover from illnesses. Equally it allows the mind to unwind, de-stress and restore mental harmony. Thus, a lack of sleep will no doubt take its toll on the individual, both mentally and physically.

Patient's Issues and Objectives	Consultation Assessment and Plan	Signature	Date	Review Date
Sleeping To promote restful sleep	1. Discuss with the patient and, or relatives, the patient's normal sleep pattern, noting any issues:			
	2. Note any past history of sleeping issues:			
	3. Note any reason, medical condition or otherwise, for any difficulty sleeping, disturbed sleep or excessive fatigue:			
	4. Note, if applicable, the name and dose of prescribed sleeping tablet, how effective it is, and when it was prescribed:			
	5. Note any safety issues, such as risk of falling, due to drowsiness caused by taking sleeping tablets:			
	6. Specify any agreed safety measures, or aids, such as bed rails required or requested by the patient. Ensure a risk assessment has been completed:			
	7. Note the patient's preferred rising time and retiring time: Rising time: .... Retiring time:			
	8. Note if these times vary and in what circumstances would they vary:			

Copyright © 2020 Planning For Care Limited

CARE PLAN: Sleeping

This care plan must be reviewed monthly (or more often if required) and each action must be signed and dated

Patient's Issues and Objectives	Consultation Assessment and Plan	Signature	Date	Review Date
	9. Note the patient's preferences regarding their ideal sleeping environment:			
	10. The temperature in the room should be comfortable for the patient. Specify ventilation, radiator setting:			
	11. Note the patient's preference regarding bed clothes and number of pillows:			
	12. Highlight how frequently the patient would like to be checked on throughout the night: | HOURLY | TWO HOURLY | THREE HOURLY | FOUR HOURLY | DOES NOT WANT TO BE DISTURBED |			
	13. Detail if the required frequency of night checks need to be assessed on a daily basis and the reason for this:			
	14. Monitor the patient throughout the night according their preference unless their physical, medical or mental condition requires more frequent checks.			
	15. Monitor the patient's sleep and liaise with the General Practitioner as necessary.			

Name	Patient/Relative Signature	Date

Copyright © 2020 Planning For Care Limited

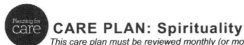

CARE PLAN: Spirituality

This care plan must be reviewed monthly (or more often if required) and each action must be signed and dated

Spirituality has been described as a desire to search for, or find, meaning and purpose in one's life, the will and reason to live, and to reflect and meditate on one's existence, which may be enhanced through art, music or literature. Religion has been described as a means of expressing spirituality through a framework of values and beliefs, often actively pursued in rituals, religious practices and reading of sacred texts. Religion might be institutionalised or informal. Restoration has been described as the ability of the spiritual dimension to positively influence the physical aspect of care.

Patient's Issues and Objectives	Consultation Assessment and Plan	Signature	Date	Review Date
Spiritual Care Respect and provide the opportunity for each individual to participate in their chosen spiritual faith and beliefs	1. Discuss with the patient and, or relative what spirituality means to them.			
	2. Note the patient's beliefs, religion or faith:			
	3. Where, through illness or incapacity or other, the patient's spiritual or religious practices have changed. Note the patient's previous practices:			
	4. Discuss with the patient and, or relative if they have any specific religious or other requests in the event of illness and record these:			
	5. Note the agreed plan of care to support the patient in practicing their chosen beliefs, religion or faith:			
	6. Discuss with the patient their wishes with regards to attending religious services.			
	7. Note any arrangements or requests:			
	8. Ensure the patient is reminded of and assisted where necessary to attend the services of their choice.			
	9. Accommodate any dietary requirements in accordance with the patient's religious beliefs and note the same:			

Copyright © 2020 Planning For Care Limited

CARE PLAN: Spirituality

This care plan must be reviewed monthly (or more often if required) and each action must be signed and dated

Patient's Issues and Objectives	Consultation Assessment and Plan	Signature	Date	Review Date
	10. Record any specific requests made known by the patient with regards to the end of life:			

Name	Patient/Relative Signature	Date

Copyright © 2020 Planning For Care Limited

CARE PLAN: Stroke (Cerebral Vascular Accident)

This care plan must be reviewed monthly (or more often if required) and each action must be signed and dated

The brain, like other organs, needs oxygen and nutrients provided by blood to function properly. A stroke, or cerebrovascular accident, CVA, occurs when the blood supply to part of the brain is disrupted or cut off, causing brain cells to die. There are two main causes, where the blood supply is stopped due to a clot, accounting for over 80% of all cases, or a weakened blood vessel supplying the brain bursts and causes a bleed. There is also a condition known as a transient ischaemic attack, TIA, where the supply of blood to the brain is temporarily interrupted, causing a mini-stroke. TIAs are often a warning sign that a stroke is coming. The symptoms following a stroke depend on the area of the brain affected, and the amount of brain tissue, which has been damaged. A stroke can result in numbness or weakness of the face, arm, or leg, especially on one side of the body, complete or partial loss of voluntary movement and/or sensation, confusion or difficulty in speaking, visual disturbance, dizziness or severe headache.

Patient's Issues and Objectives	Consultation Assessment and Plan	Signature	Date	Review Date
Stroke (Cerebral Vascular Accident) To maintain an optimal level of independence and lifestyle	1. Discuss the condition with the patient and, or relative and agree the plan of care.			
	2. Note the patient's and, or relative's understanding of the condition and any concerns or anxieties they have:			
	3. Note the patient's past history if available:			
	4. Highlight any of the symptoms of stroke experienced by the patient: | SEVERE HEADACHE | WEAKNESS OF THE FACE | UNABLE TO SMILE | MOUTH HAS DROPPED | NUMBNESS | | DIZZINESS | SUDDEN CONFUSION | WEAKNESS OF AN ARM | WEAKNESS OF A LEG | DIFFICULTY WALKING | | LOSS OF VOLUNTARY MOVEMENTS | DIFFICULTY SPEAKING | OTHER............			
	5. Note how the stroke has affected the patient emotionally, and physically, the side and areas of the body affected:			
	6. Note the agreed plan of care to address any issues the patient has with any of the activities of daily living:			

Copyright © 2020 Planning For Care Limited

CARE PLAN: Stroke (Cerebral Vascular Accident)

This care plan must be reviewed monthly (or more often if required) and each action must be signed and dated

Patient's Issues and Objectives	Consultation Assessment and Plan	Signature	Date	Review Date
	7. Highlight any specialised equipment that may assist the patient: | ANTI SPILLAGE CUP | ADAPTED CUTLERY | NON SLIP TABLE MATS | PLATE GUARD | MECHANICAL HELPING HAND | | WALKING AID |...			
	8. Outline if the level of care required varies on a day to day basis and the reason:			
	9. Note the prescribed medication, dose and frequency:			
	10. Liaise with the General Practitioner as necessary.			
	.... (blank lines)			

Name	Patient/Relative Signature	Date

Copyright © 2020 Planning For Care Limited

CARE PLAN: Ulcerative Colitis
This care plan must be reviewed monthly (or more often if required) and each action must be signed and dated

Ulcerative colitis is an inflammatory bowel disease, which causes long-lasting inflammation and ulcers in the digestive tract. It is a long-term chronic condition with symptoms usually developing over time, rather than suddenly. It can be debilitating and sometimes can lead to life-threatening complications such as bowel cancer or primary sclerosing cholangitis. While it has no known cure, treatment can greatly reduce the effects of the disease and even bring about long-term remission. The exact cause of ulcerative colitis is unknown, although it is thought to be the result of a problem with the immune system. It is thought that the immune system mistakes harmless bacteria inside the colon for a threat and attacks the tissues of the colon, causing it to become inflamed.

Patient's Issues and Objectives	Consultation Assessment and Plan	Signature	Date	Review Date
Ulcerative Colitis To regain normal bowel function and promote effective management	1. Discuss the condition with the patient and, or relative and agree the plan of care.			
	2. Note the patient's and, or relative's understanding of the condition and any concerns or anxieties they have:			
	3. Note the past medical history of the bowel condition, when it was diagnosed, and treatments prescribed:			
	4. Highlight the symptoms experienced by the patient: | RECURRING DIARRHOEA | ABDOMINAL PAIN | NEEDING TO EMPTY BOWELS FREQUENTLY | LOSS OF APPETITE | | WEIGHT LOSS | FATIGUE |............			
	5. Highlight the symptoms experienced by the patient during a flare up of the disease: | DEHYDRATION | SWOLLEN JOINTS | MOUTH ULCERS | AREAS OF PAINFUL SKIN | RED SKIN | SWOLLEN SKIN | | IRRITATED EYES |............			
	6. Note the patient's normal bowel function: Frequency: Time of day:			
	7. Note the prescribed medication, dosage and frequency:			
	8. Encourage sufficient fluid intake 1500mls- 2000mls per day. Note if there are issues with fluid intake and specify any assistance required:			

Copyright © 2020 Planning For Care Limited

CARE PLAN: Ulcerative Colitis

This care plan must be reviewed monthly (or more often if required) and each action must be signed and dated

Patient's Issues and Objectives	Consultation Assessment and Plan	Signature	Date	Review Date
	9. Detail any issues the patient has with the activities of daily living, due to the condition, and the agreed plan to address them:			
	10. Observe for any of the following signs or symptoms of complications, if present consult the patient's General Practitioner: • Osteoporosis • Primary sclerosing cholangitis where the bile ducts become progressively inflamed and damaged • Toxic megacolon, where gas is trapped causing the colon to swell • Septicaemia • Bowel cancer			
	....			

Name	Patient/Relative Signature	Date

Copyright © 2020 Planning For Care Limited

CARE PLAN: Underactive Thyroid

This care plan must be reviewed monthly (or more often if required) and each action must be signed and dated

The thyroid produces a hormone called thyroxine, which controls how much energy the body uses. When the thyroid does not produce enough thyroxine many of the body's functions slow down. An Underactive thyroid cannot be prevented. Most cases of underactive thyroid are caused either by the immune system attacking the thyroid or a damaged thyroid. An underactive thyroid is a life-long condition and the treatment is to take thyroxine. Levothyroxine does not usually have any side effects as the tablets simply replace a missing hormone.

Patient's Issues and Objectives	Consultation Assessment and Plan	Signature	Date	Review Date
Underactive thyroid To maintain thyroxine levels within normal limits	1. Discuss the condition with the patient and, or relatives and agree plan of care.			
	2. Note the patient's and, or relatives understanding of the condition and any concerns or anxieties they have:			
	3. Note when the condition was diagnosed and the treatment received:			
	4. Highlight any symptoms experienced by the patient: | SENSITIVE TO COLD | WEIGHT GAIN | CONSTIPATION | DEPRESSION | TIREDNESS | DRY AND SCALY SKIN | | SLOWNESS OF THE BODY AND MIND | MUSCLE ACHES AND WEAKNESS | MUSCLE CRAMPS | BRITTLE NAILS |			
	5. Note the prescribed medication, dose and frequency:			
	6. Observe for signs and symptoms of changes in levels of thyroxine.			
	7. Obtain bloods for routine thyroxine levels annually unless the General Practitioner requests more frequently and record the results in the patient's notes.			
	8. Liaise with the General Practitioner as required.			

Copyright © 2020 Planning For Care Limited

CARE PLAN: Underactive Thyroid

This care plan must be reviewed monthly (or more often if required) and each action must be signed and dated

Patient 's Issues and Objectives	Consultation Assessment and Plan	Signature	Date	Review Date

Name	Patient /Relative Signature	Date

Copyright © 2020 Planning For Care Limited

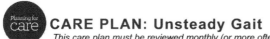

CARE PLAN: Unsteady Gait

This care plan must be reviewed monthly (or more often if required) and each action must be signed and dated

Gait abnormalities or unsteadiness is a common complaint, one third of elderly people experience difficulties with walking. An unsteady gait can be caused by a disease of, or damage to the legs and feet including the bones, joints, blood vessels, muscles, and other soft tissues or to the nervous system that controls the movements necessary for walking. An unsteady gait may occur as a result of a temporary condition, such as an injury or infection, or it may indicate a long-term, chronic problem. When unsteadiness is related to a sprain, strain, or minor injury, analgesic and anti-inflammatory medications may be effective for relief. More severe injuries and conditions require specific therapies that are directed at the underlying cause of the problem.

Patient's Issues and Objectives	Consultation Assessment and Plan	Signature	Date	Review Date
Unsteady gait **Risk of falling** **To promote a safe environment and minimise the risk of falling**	1. Discuss the issue with the patient and, or relative and agree the plan of care.			
	2. Complete a falls risk assessment and discuss with the patient and, or relative any factors causing an increased risk of falls. Note any concerns or anxieties they have:			
	3. Note the cause of the unsteady gait, such as medical condition, injury or infection, if known:			
	4. Note if the patient has any issues with their memory or understanding:			
	5. Note any medication which may affect the patient's unsteadiness:			
	6. Highlight the agreed plan of care: <ul><li>ensure the environment is free from obstacles and obstructions</li><li>ensure the patient's buzzer is within reach</li><li>where the patient has impaired eyesight encourage them to wear prescribed glasses</li><li>where the patient has impaired hearing encourage them to wear their hearing aid</li><li>ensure the patient's room is well lit</li><li>encourage the patient to wear suitable, well-fitting footwear</li><li>ensure the patient has a raised toilet seat</li><li>review medication</li></ul>			

Copyright © 2020 Planning For Care Limited

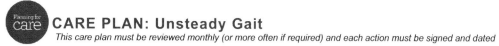

CARE PLAN: Unsteady Gait

This care plan must be reviewed monthly (or more often if required) and each action must be signed and dated

Patient's Issues and Objectives	Consultation Assessment and Plan	Signature	Date	Review Date
	7. Note the agreed plan of care for mobilising, or addressing any issues regarding the patient's safety:			
	8. Highlight if a form of restraint has been assessed as beneficial to the patient and agreed as part of the plan of care: | PRESSURE MAT | LAP STRAP | SPECIALISED CHAIR | BED RAILS |			
	9. Ensure all equipment is routinely checked to be safe and in good working order, such as walking aids, wheelchairs, commodes and arm chairs.			
	10. Review the falls risk assessment monthly and review the care plan accordingly.			
	11. Where the patient has had more than one fall, consider commencing a falls diary to identify the times of the day and the circumstances of any fall.			
	12. Liaise with the patient's General Practitioner where appropriate.			

Name	Patient/Relative Signature	Date

Copyright © 2020 Planning For Care Limited

CARE PLAN: Urinary Incontinence

This care plan must be reviewed monthly (or more often if required) and each action must be signed and dated

Urinary incontinence is the inability to control the bladder, and the unintentional passing of urine, causing urine to leak unexpectedly. It is a common and often embarrassing problem. The severity of urinary incontinence ranges from occasionally leaking urine when exercising, heavy lifting, coughing, or sneezing, to having no control at all.

Patient's Issues and Objectives	Consultation Assessment and Plan	Signature	Date	Review Date
Urinary Incontinence **To promote continence where possible** **To effectively manage the condition**	**1. Discuss the condition with the patient and, or relative and agree the plan of care.**			
	2. Note the patient's and, or the relative's understanding of the condition and any concerns or anxieties they have:			
	3. Note any past history of urinary continence issues:			
	4. Complete a continence assessment.			
	5. Highlight the symptoms experienced by the patient: | URINARY FREQUENCY | URINARY HESITANCY | URINARY URGENCY | NO SENSATION OF NEEDING TO URINATE | | DRIBBLING AFTER PASSING URINE | POOR URINARY STREAM | NEEDING TO PASS URINE DURING THE NIGHT | | STRESS INCONTINENCE | NEW ONSET INCONTINENCE DURING THE NIGHT | OVER FLOW INCONTINENCE |			
	6. Highlight any contributing factors: | DISORIENTATION | CONFUSION | DEMENTIA | PSYCHOLOGICAL PROBLEMS | | POOR MOBILITY | USES A WALKING AID | IMMOBILITY | POOR DEXTERITY | NEEDS HELP UNDRESSING |			
	7. Specify the agreed plan of care to assist with, or improve any of the contributing factors:			
	8. Specify the agreed plan of care based on outcome of the patient's continence assessment: **Day:**............ .... **Night:**			

Copyright © 2020 Planning For Care Limited

CARE PLAN: Urinary Incontinence

This care plan must be reviewed monthly (or more often if required) and each action must be signed and dated

Patient's Issues and Objectives	Consultation Assessment and Plan	Signature	Date	Review Date
	9. Note any prescribed containment products:			
	10. Note any prescribed medication to assist continence, the dose and frequency:			
	11. Encourage adequate fluid intake1500 - 2000mls, explaining the importance of this.			
	12. Note if the patient has any issues taking an adequate fluid intake and the agreed plan to address this:			
	13. Observe skin integrity and maintain excellent personal hygiene standards.			
	14. Liaise with the patients General Practitioner as required.			

Name	Patient/Relative Signature	Date

Copyright © 2020 Planning For Care Limited

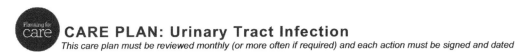

CARE PLAN: Urinary Tract Infection

This care plan must be reviewed monthly (or more often if required) and each action must be signed and dated

A Urinary Tract Infection, UTI, is a bacterial infection that affects any part of the urinary tract. Symptoms include frequently feeling the need and, or an actual need to urinate, pain during urination, strong smelling urine and cloudy urine. The main causal agent is Escherichia coli. Although urine contains a variety of fluids, salts and waste products it does not usually have bacteria in it, but when bacteria gets into the bladder or kidney, the bacteria may multiply in the urine and may cause a Urinary Tract Infection. Urine is normally sterile, and the normal flow of urine usually prevents bacteria from growing in the urinary tract. When urine stays in the bladder, however bacteria have a chance to grow and infect the urinary tract.

Patient's Issues and Objectives	Consultation Assessment and Plan	Signature	Date	Review Date
Urinary Tract Infection **Treat infection and reduce risk of infection re-occurring**	1. Discuss the condition with the patient and, or relatives and agree the plan of care.			
	2. Note any concerns or anxieties they have:			
	3. Note any history of previous urinary tract infections:			
	4. Highlight which of the following signs and symptoms the patient is experiencing: | FREQUENTLY FEELING THE NEED TO URINATE | FREQUENTLY PASSING URINE | FOUL SMELLING URINE | | CLOUDY URINE | UNCHARACTERISTIC CONFUSION | INCREASED CONFUSION | PAIN IN LOWER ABDOMEN |			
	5. Obtain a urine sample for multi stick urinalysis and note the result:			
	6. Where the multi stick urinalysis shows an abnormality, obtain a mid stream specimen of urine (MSSU) and send to the laboratory for analysis. Note date MSSU sent:			
	7. Consult the patient's General Practitioner for advice.			
	8. Note the prescribed medication, dose and frequency:			
	9. Discuss the importance of taking an adequate fluid intake 1500-2000mls daily and encourage this.			
	10. Note if there are any issues the patient has drinking adequate fluids and the agreed care plan to improve this:			

Copyright © 2020 Planning For Care Limited

CARE PLAN: Urinary Tract Infection

This care plan must be reviewed monthly (or more often if required) and each action must be signed and dated

Patient's Issues and Objectives	Consultation Assessment and Plan	Signature	Date	Review Date
	11. Note if dehydration is an issue and commence a fluid balance chart to monitor intake and output:			
	12. Note the patient's preferences for fluids:			
	13. Four days after completion of the course of antibiotics a further MSSU must be sent to the laboratory and the results must be recorded in the patient's notes.			
	14. Liaise with the General Practitioner as necessary.			

Name	Patient/Relative Signature	Date

Copyright © 2020 Planning For Care Limited

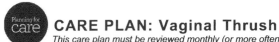

CARE PLAN: Vaginal Thrush

This care plan must be reviewed monthly (or more often if required) and each action must be signed and dated

Most women experience occasional bouts of a common yeast infection known as vaginal thrush. It causes itching, irritation and swelling of the vagina and surrounding area, sometimes with a creamy white cottage cheese-like discharge. Vaginal thrush is fairly harmless but it can be uncomfortable and it can keep coming back, which is known as recurrent thrush. Thrush is more likely in pregnancy, or as a result of taking antibiotics, or diabetes or a weakened immune system.

Patient's Issues And Objectives	Consultation Assessment and Plan	Signature	Date	Review Date
Vaginal Thrush To promote recovery and minimise discomfort	1. Discuss the condition with the patient and, or relative and agree the plan of care.			
	2. Note the patient's and, or relative's understanding of the condition and any concerns or anxieties they have:			
	3. Note any past history of thrush and the treatment prescribed:			
	4. Highlight and discuss with the patient and/or the relatives any possible contributing factors: | ANTIBIOTIC THERAPY | DIABETES | WEAKENED IMMUNE SYSTEM |			
	5. Highlight the symptoms experienced by the patient: | VAGINAL ITCH OR IRRITATION | SWELLING OF THE VAGINA AND SURROUNDING AREA | | CREAMY WHITE DISCHARGE "COTTAGE CHEESE LIKE" | STINGING SENSATION WHEN URINATING | OTHER:			
	6. Consult with the patient's General Practitioner.			
	7. Note the prescribed medication, dosage, and treatment regime:			
	8. Note any issues the patient has with the treatment and the agreed plan of care to address them:			
	9. Monitor the condition and liaise with the patient's General Practitioner as required.			

Copyright © 2020 Planning For Care Limited

CARE PLAN: Vaginal Thrush

This care plan must be reviewed monthly (or more often if required) and each action must be signed and dated

Patient's Issues And Objectives	Consultation Assessment and Plan	Signature	Date	Review Date

Name	Patient /Relative Signature	Date

Copyright © 2020 Planning For Care Limited

CARE PLAN: Validation and Memory Aids

This care plan must be reviewed monthly (or more often if required) and each action must be signed and dated

In the early stages of dementia, memory aids such as lists, diaries, clocks and clear written instructions can help jog the patient's memory if they are willing and able to make use of them. A memory aid may be a written summary or outline of important details, which can calm a patient who has dementia or memory issues. Another aid might be a topic of conversation, or something the patient loves, or is important to them. Validation Therapy advocates that, rather than trying to bring the person with dementia back to reality, it can be more positive and beneficial to enter their reality. In this way empathy is developed, building trust and a sense of security. This in turn reduces anxiety.

Patient's Issues and Objectives	Consultation Assessment and Plan	Signature	Date	Review Date
Memory Impairment To calm, comfort and alleviate anxiety, minimise agitation and minimise distress	1. Consult with relatives and other health professionals and detail all involved in the consultation:			
	2. Specify what time, or stage of the patient's life, the patient believes he or she is at?			
	3. What in the past has had a calming effect or influence on the patient, in terms of the environment, music, or touch?			
	4. What topics of conversation, or things can stimulate, uplift, or improve the mood of the patient?			

Copyright © 2020 Planning For Care Limited

CARE PLAN: Validation and Memory Aids

This care plan must be reviewed monthly (or more often if required) and each action must be signed and dated

Patient's Issues and Objectives	Consultation Assessment and Plan	Signature	Date	Review Date
	5. Detail any phrases, subjects, or topics of conversation or things, which can calm the patient:			

Name	Patient/Relative Signature	Date

Copyright © 2020 Planning For Care Limited

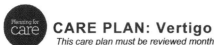

CARE PLAN: Vertigo

This care plan must be reviewed monthly (or more often if required) and each action must be signed and dated

Vertigo is a symptom, rather than a condition itself. It is the sensation or feeling that a person can experience, that they themselves, or the environment around them, is moving or spinning. This feeling may be barely noticeable, or it may be so severe that they find it difficult to keep their balance and do everyday tasks. Attacks of vertigo can develop suddenly and last for a few seconds, or they may last much longer. Severe vertigo, may be constant and last for several days, making normal life very difficult. Other symptoms associated with vertigo may include loss of balance, which can make it difficult to stand or walk, feeling sick, or being sick and suffering from dizziness. Vertigo is commonly caused by a problem with the way balance works in the inner ear, although it can also be caused by problems in certain parts of the brain.

Patient's Issues and Objectives	Consultation Assessment and Plan	Signature	Date	Review Date
Vertigo To manage and minimise the symptoms of vertigo	1. Discuss the condition with the patient and, or relative and agree the plan of care.			
	2. Note the patient's and, or relative's understanding of the condition and any concerns or anxieties they have:			
	3. Note the past history of when vertigo was diagnosed and the cause if known:			
	4. Highlight the symptoms experienced by the patient: | LOSS OF BALANCE | NAUSEA | VOMITING | DIZZINESS | SPECIFY:			
	5. Note the prescribed medication, dose and frequency:			
	6. Highlight the agreed plan of care to minimise the effects of vertigo: • encourage simple exercises • encourage the patient to sleep with his or her head slightly raised using extra pillows • advise the patient to get up slowly when getting out of bed and to sit on the edge of the bed for a minute or so before standing • encourage the patient to avoid bending down to pick up items • encourage the patient to avoid extending their neck, by looking up • encourage the patient to move their head carefully and slowly during daily activities • encourage the patient to do exercises which trigger the vertigo, so that their brain becomes more used to the sensation and reduces the symptoms			

Copyright © 2020 Planning For Care Limited

CARE PLAN: Vertigo

This care plan must be reviewed monthly (or more often if required) and each action must be signed and dated

Patient's Issues and Objectives	Consultation Assessment and Plan	Signature	Date	Review Date
	7. If the patient is a high risk of falling, detail any agreed safety measures which are in place:			
	8. Liaise with the General Practitioner as required.			

Name	Patient/Relative Signature	Date

Copyright © 2020 Planning For Care Limited

CARE PLAN: Visual Impairment

This care plan must be reviewed monthly (or more often if required) and each action must be signed and dated

If a person is visually impaired, they will have some loss of vision or some distortion to their vision. Depending on the severity of sight loss or the degree of distortion, the conditions are usually referred to as partial sightedness or blindness. Visual impairment, which can't be treated can be difficult to come to terms with. Some people go through a process similar to bereavement, where they experience a range of emotions including shock, anger, and denial, before eventually coming to accept their condition. Causes of visual impairment include, cataracts where a cloudy area forms in the lens of the eye, glaucoma where fluid in the eye cannot drain properly and there is a build up of pressure which results in damage to the optic nerve, age related macular degeneration where the vision gradually deteriorates with age, and diabetic retinopathy where the tiny blood vessels that nourish the retina become damaged.

Patient's Issues and Objectives	Consultation Assessment and Plan	Signature	Date	Review Date
Impaired Sight To maximise sight and reduce potential risks	1. Discuss the condition with the patient and, or relative and agree the plan of care.			
	2. Note the patient's and, or relative's understanding of the condition and any concerns and anxieties they have:			
	3. Highlight the cause if known: | GLAUCOMA | CATARACTS | MACULAR DEGENERATION | AGE RELATED |			
	4. Highlight the degree of visual impairment: | REGISTERED BLIND | PARTIALLY SIGHTED | POOR WITH GLASSES | | GOOD WITH GLASSES |...			
	5. Highlight any contributing factors: | OBESITY | SMOKING | DIABETES TYPE 1 | DIABETES TYPE 2 | KIDNEY DISEASE | EXCESSIVE ALCOHOL | | EXCESSIVE SALT | LACK OF EXERCISE | MEDICATION, STEROIDS |			
	6. Note the past history of visual impairment and any treatment received:			
	7. Detail any issues the patient has with the activities of daily living as a result of being visually impaired, and the agreed plan to address them:...			

Copyright © 2020 Planning For Care Limited

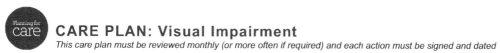

CARE PLAN: Visual Impairment

This care plan must be reviewed monthly (or more often if required) and each action must be signed and dated

Patient's Issues and Objectives	Consultation Assessment and Plan	Signature	Date	Review Date
	8. Highlight any aids which may assist the patient, or improve his or her quality of life: | PLATE GUARDS | SPECIALISED CUTLERY | NON SLIP MAT FOR PLATE | MAGNIFYING GLASS | MUSIC SYSTEM | | RADIO | TALKING BOOK | TALKING NEWSPAPER | OTHER:			
	9. Detail any issues the patient has with safety due to being visually impaired, and the agreed plan to address them:			
	10. Note, where appropriate, the prescribed eye drops, dose and frequency:			
	11. Specify any issues the patient has with wearing glasses:			
	12. Monitor the condition on an ongoing basis, and report any change in eyesight, or discomfort of eyes and refer to ophthalmologist immediately. Arrange an annual eye test and examination.			

Name	Patient/Relative Signature	Date

Copyright © 2020 Planning For Care Limited

CARE PLAN: Warfarin Therapy

This care plan must be reviewed monthly (or more often if required) and each action must be signed and dated

Warfarin medication is used to treat blood clots, such as deep vein thrombosis or pulmonary embolus, and, or prevent new clots from forming in the body. Preventing harmful blood clots helps to reduce the risk of a stroke or heart attack. Conditions that increase the risk of developing blood clots include a certain type of irregular heart rhythm called atrial fibrillation, heart valve replacement, recent heart attack, and certain surgeries such as fracture and hip/knee replacement. Warfarin is commonly called a "blood thinner", but the more correct term for it is an "anticoagulant". The blood needs vitamin K to be able to clot. Warfarin slows the production of vitamin K in the body, which increases the time it takes for the blood to clot. It helps the blood to flow freely around the body and prevents any clots forming in the heart or in the blood vessels. While taking warfarin, the dose will be monitored using the international normalisation ratio, INR, which measures how long it takes the blood to clot. Many herbal medicines and supplements can interact with warfarin, it is important to check with the anticoagulant clinic, GP or pharmacist. Aspirin and Ibuprofen should not be taken when taking warfarin.

Patient's Issues and Objectives	Consultation Assessment and Plan	Signature	Date	Review Date
Warfarin therapy To maintain the patient's blood clotting levels at an optimum level following tests for International Normalised Ratio	1. Discuss with the patient and, or relatives the medication and therapy and agree the plan of care.			
	2. Note the patient and, or relatives understanding of the treatment and any anxieties or concerns they may have:			
	3. Explain that the warfarin dosage can frequently vary, as it is based on keeping the blood clotting factor level between 2 and 3, and external factors can cause variations in these levels leading to frequent changes in dosage.			
	4. Advise that an increase in analgesia or antibiotics therapy can cause the blood clotting factor levels to change.			
	5. Advise the patient to avoid taking any cranberry juice, cranberries, or products containing cranberries as it affects the warfarin therapy			
	6. Note the patient's past medical history and the reason for anticoagulant therapy:			
	7. Note the patient's International Normalised Ratio results in their notes and Medical Administration Records sheet.			
	8. Explain that the anticoagulant nurse routinely takes blood to check International Normalised Ratio levels and that the frequency of blood tests can change according to the stability of the results.			
	9. Keep the patient and, or relative updated with blood results and warfarin levels, if appropriate.			

Copyright © 2020 Planning For Care Limited

CARE PLAN: Warfarin Therapy

This care plan must be reviewed monthly (or more often if required) and each action must be signed and dated

Patient's Issues and Objectives	Consultation Assessment and Plan	Signature	Date	Review Date
	10. Observe for side effects of anticoagulant therapy and highlight any experienced: \ \ | SEVERE BLEEDING | SEVERE BRUISING | COUGHING UP BLOOD | VOMITING UP BLOOD | BLEEDING GUMS | \ | NOSE BLEEDS LASTING MORE THAN 10 MINS | BLACK STOOLS | HEADACHES | BLEEDING FROM THE RECTUM | \ | BLEEDING FROM THE VAGINA |..			
	11. Liaise with the patient's General Practitioner as necessary.			

Name	Patient/Relative Signature	Date

Copyright © 2020 Planning For Care Limited

Printed in Great Britain
by Amazon